Pioneers In Scrubs

Nursing In A Tech Age

By

Zawadi Nkulikwa

Preface

In *Pioneers in Scrubs: Nursing in a Tech Age*, we explore the ever-evolving landscape of modern healthcare. This journey is narrated through the lives of compelling individuals at the forefront of transformation. Every chapter of this book provides a unique perspective on the current state of nursing, offering readers valuable insight into the dynamic field.

As a writer, I am deeply intrigued by the intersection of science, religion, and imagination, and I have incorporated these elements into the lives of my characters. Their personal experiences mirror our progress in this modern age, marked by the merging of compassion and technological innovation.

We will encounter individuals like Emma, who grapples with integrating artificial intelligence in healthcare, and David, whose work is impacted by global health challenges. Each of these individuals is introduced to us chapter by chapter. The collective experiences of these individuals and their colleagues provide a compelling portrayal of the difficulties and accomplishments faced in a rapidly evolving industry.

Indeed, this book may be classified as a work of fiction; however, it is firmly rooted in the realities of nursing in the contemporary world. It takes inspiration from numerous real-life nurses and healthcare professionals who have been trailblazers, navigating the challenges of technology-driven healthcare with compassion and determination.

I am confident that *Pioneers in Scrubs* will engage your imagination and deepen your appreciation for the often-overlooked individuals in the healthcare industry. This aims to recognise and appreciate the individuals who wear scrubs, embrace technological advancements, and face each day with courage and a mind filled with creative ideas.

We warmly welcome a world where every heartbeat holds great importance, every technological advancement carries weight, and every nurse's story is a source of inspiration in the contemporary era of healthcare.

Acknowledgements

I am thankful for the Divine grace and inspiration that have guided me through the complex realm of School Nursing. This journey, marked by faith and determination, showcases a solid dedication to service and education. I am grateful for the Guiding Light that has led me to fulfil my purpose with commitment and understanding.

I want to thank Mrs. Bibiana Mwaluko, the former Dean, for recognising my potential to influence nursing education positively. Your trust in my abilities and consistent support have empowered me and set the stage for ongoing achievements with the current Dean, Ms. Rachel Masibo. You have created a nurturing environment at the School of Nursing and St. John's University of Tanzania that encourages academic and personal development.

Maria Simbowe, my life's rock, and our beloved children, Vahid, Zenobia, Navid, and Roshanak, your unwavering support and understanding have been my anchor throughout this critical project. Your kindness and the deep connection we have are truly invaluable.

I admire Prof. Casmir Rubagumya's deep expertise and unwavering enthusiasm for languages and literature. Your help and encouragement have played a crucial role in moulding my work. Your insights have significantly impacted my manuscript, and I genuinely appreciate your assistance.

Dr. Safari Mafu, my esteemed mentor and leader, your steadfast support and motivation were essential in finishing this project. Your guidance has illuminated the path towards our shared objective. My brother, Godfrey William, your dedication to thorough analysis and insightful viewpoints have consistently motivated and amazed me, encouraging me to delve deeper into the quest for knowledge.

I am thankful to my current and former St. John's University students and the teachers and staff who have significantly impacted my growth. The interactions and shared moments of discovery have been priceless, underscoring the significance of our collaborative efforts.

Pioneers in Scrubs: Nursing in a Tech Age highlights the combined efforts of everyone involved in this project. This book combines our collective experiences, hopes, and explorations in the constantly changing nursing field. I want to thank all of you for participating in this incredible adventure. This book aims to provide readers with a wealth of knowledge, inspiration, and a deep understanding of the nursing profession's dedication to excellence, compassion, and creativity.

We appreciate and admire your thoughtfulness.

Prologue

There is a realm where the essence of humanity and the marvel of technology harmoniously intertwine. This domain is nestled in the heart of a bustling city beneath the constant radiance of vibrant neon lights. Our story unfolds within the corridors of a hospital widely recognised for its remarkable achievements in human perseverance and scientific brilliance.

Aside from its focus on medical professionals, *Pioneers in Scrubs: Nursing in a Technological Age* provides a broader perspective beyond the narrative of nurses. It is a journey of the human mind navigating the intricate interplay of technology and the timeless art of caring for others. Within these pages, you will have the chance to meet Emma, whose skills extend from mastering touchscreens to providing comfort to the unwell. Emma embodies the modern era that nursing has entered. The aspirations that David has set for himself are just as audacious as the global health issues that he is currently confronting.

Each chapter is a captivating tapestry that intertwines the stories of individuals donning scrubs throughout the book. Their diverse experiences, including Lina's innovative teaching methods, Aisha's commitment to promoting inclusivity, Miriam's ethical dilemmas in the era of AI, and Zara's impressive rise in healthcare leadership, form the foundation of a compelling and interconnected story.

John's quiet struggle with mental health, Grace's passionate advocacy for older people, Noah's battle with burnout, and Sophia's pursuit of equity highlight the many pressing issues in modern nursing.

As you delve into these pages, you will embark on a voyage encompassing the digital realm, the human element, the worldwide scope, and the individual obstacles. This novel aims beyond mere storytelling, presenting a rich tapestry that intertwines human experience, technological advancements, and the ceaseless nature of change. Join us for an invitation to witness the dawn of a new era in nursing, where every heartbeat becomes a testament to strength, and every breakthrough brings us closer to a more empathetic world.

Welcome to *Pioneers in Scrubs: Nursing in a Tech Age*. Here, we embrace the intersection of healthcare and technology, where the dedication and compassion of those who nurture life's most fragile aspects shape the future.

CHAPTER 1

Care's Changing Face

The Mercy Mwongozo Hospital stood tall in the heart of the bustling metropolis, symbolising the ever-evolving nature of progress. Surrounded by buildings that resonated with the aspirations of humanity, it served as a testament to our collective drive for advancement. The glass exterior, reflecting the morning sunlight, contained tales of human experience, adversity, and the unwavering determination of those who chose to overcome.

Emma's fingers glided across the touchscreen, her eyes swiftly taking in the vibrant visuals displaying the essential information. She was consistently amazed by the intersection of technology and healthcare. The steady hum of equipment blended harmoniously with the distant chatter of her colleagues, creating a captivating symphony of modern medicine in action. She pondered how nursing had evolved from traditional bedside care to a current field where technology was crucial alongside compassionate client care.

David carefully adjusted his headset, readying himself for a video appointment with a client in a distant community on the other side of the globe. He pondered how the world had become more minor, yet the health disparities had become even more glaring. His career, once confined to the hospital, has now expanded to distant corners of the world, surpassing insurmountable barriers.

An experienced nurse and instructor, Lina quickly skimmed through a computerised textbook on advanced genomics in another part of the hospital, her mind filled with endless possibilities. She saw great potential in these pages, envisioning a future where nurses would transcend their traditional roles as carers and become pioneers and influencers in healthcare. Her unwavering dedication to integrating these advancements into her curriculum matched her deep devotion to her students.

Aisha strolled through the bustling streets of the diverse neighbourhood surrounding the hospital, focusing on the clients she would be attending today. Every individual brought a unique blend of cultural and social experiences, presenting a complex challenge beyond therapy. She had a responsibility that went beyond simply administering drugs - she needed to understand, value, and connect with different cultures. According to her perspective, nursing encompasses clinical expertise and cultural competence.

As the city awoke to a new day, these nurses were each contributing to the ever-evolving healthcare landscape. Their separate yet interconnected paths showcased a profession changing—a shift driven by technology, confronted by global inequalities, enhanced by cultural diversity, and rooted in enduring values of empathy and understanding. As a microcosm of this evolving world, Mercy Mwongozo served as a centre of healing, a beacon of optimism, and a messenger of a fresh era in nursing.

As the day passed, Miriam, who worked in the hospital's advanced wing, faced a common dilemma in his industry. On the screens before him, complex algorithms and client data were displayed, representing the advanced tools of modern medicine that hold the potential for extended and improved lives. Despite every advancement, Miriam faced the moral dilemma of prolonging life while sacrificing its quality. His work had expanded beyond conventional nursing, encompassing bioethics and client advocacy in an era where technology often surpassed ethical considerations.

Zara, meantime, was fully engaged in a dynamic policy meeting, her voice filled with enthusiasm and determination. She had transcended the confines of hospital rooms, taking her fight for improved healthcare policies to the corridors of influence. Every statement she made showcased her evolution from a practical nurse to a determined champion, shaping laws that would shape the future of healthcare while guaranteeing its availability and compassion.

John, another nurse whose path had taken a different direction, sat at a support group for healthcare professionals in a more tranquil part of town. He discovered solace and meaning in this place, surrounded by fellow individuals who openly shared their struggles. The cognitive strain of nursing, frequently overlooked due to the physical demands, was now becoming evident. Having experienced his battles with mental health, John has emerged as a beacon of hope, advocating for support systems and promoting awareness surrounding the well-being of carers.

Grace spent the evening visiting one of her elderly clients at their home. Grace adeptly navigated the challenges posed by the ageing population by combining time-honoured nursing techniques with cutting-edge senior care practices. Her composed demeanour and deep understanding of her client's needs reflected an aspect of nursing that no technology can replicate - the essential human touch, empathy, and connection at the core of healthcare.

As the sun dipped below the horizon, these nurses bore the weight of the day's triumphs and sorrows. Their narratives transcended mere personal anecdotes, weaving together to form a larger fabric reflecting a vocation's profound evolution. They were part of a broader movement reshaping the nursing concept in a world where care was as varied and ever-changing as the individuals it catered to, spanning hospitals and residences, policy chambers, and far-flung corners connected through digital networks. With its bustling corridors and the constant hum of activity, Mercy Mwongozo embodied a microcosm of the vast, complex, and ever-evolving world of nursing.

Noah completed his extensive shift beneath the sparkling night sky, the hospital lights gradually dimming as he ventured into the chilly evening. However, his thoughts remained confined within the boundaries of the wards. The day's events lingered, mirroring his deepening worry about nursing burnout, a topic that had sparked his growing interest. Noah's nursing career had shown him that prioritising the well-being of others often took a toll on one's physical and mental health. The burden of responsibility, the emotional toll, and the relentless pace had all led him to advocate for a cause steadily gaining momentum: the well-being of healthcare providers.

Sophia was engaged in a spirited discussion with community leaders in another part of town. Her focus had shifted from the hospital to the broader realm of public health, specifically in underserved communities where healthcare access was intertwined with social justice and not just medical care. Her days were filled with challenges, like finding funding for local health projects and creating programs tailored to the unique needs of different populations. Sophia's work showcased the evolving role of nurses as catalysts for change in the pursuit of health equity, going beyond their traditional caregiving responsibilities.

With the break of dawn, these nurses, each facing their challenges and triumphs, felt a renewed sense of determination. They were pioneers of a new era in healthcare, where a deeper understanding of the principles of healing and compassion complemented expertise in the field.

Emma pondered the remarkable technological advancements that had transformed her profession entirely as she embarked on her next shift. Although she could access advanced computerised instruments for unparalleled precision and efficiency in client care, she always maintained a personal touch. Her interactions with clients were characterised by a deep sense of compassion and comprehension despite the frequent reliance on screens and technology. According to her perspective, the core of nursing remained the connection between nurse and client, with technology serving as a valuable tool to enhance, but not substitute for, this bond.

Meanwhile, David continued his dedicated efforts to address the global health disparities. His telehealth visits with clients in rural places went beyond mere consultations; they served as vital connections, linking underprivileged communities with essential healthcare services they would otherwise lack. His work was a constant reminder of healthcare disparities and the nurses' crucial role in addressing these disparities. For David, each client served as a poignant reminder of the interconnectedness of global health. It highlighted the profound impact that a nurse in one part of the world can have on saving the life of someone thousands of miles away.

The fast-paced world of academia consumed Lina's day as she worked to integrate the latest scientific breakthroughs into the nursing curriculum. She passionately believed that future nurses should receive comprehensive education, encompassing technical skills and ethical and emotional development, to tackle the upcoming challenges effectively. Her classrooms were spaces where deep thinking and empathy thrived side by side. Aisha's commitment to fostering inclusivity and understanding shines through her community engagement programs. Her work was based on the belief that comprehensive healthcare necessitated an appreciation for cultural intricacies alongside medical expertise. She advocated for the importance of cultural competency in nursing education, emphasising the need for future nurses to be well-prepared to care for diverse clients.

Miriam found himself deeply engaged in the forefront of debates surrounding the utilisation of AI in healthcare as he sought to strike a delicate balance between technological advancements and ethical considerations. His perspectives, acquired through his firsthand experiences and understanding of medical ethics, were pivotal in shaping technology integration policies in client care. Miriam emphasised the importance of carefully weighing the benefits of technology in improving lives while also considering the need to maintain the human aspect of healthcare.

Zara's exploration of health policy demanded that she navigate the intricate interplay of politics, economics, and healthcare. Through her advocacy work, she gained firsthand experience of the complex dynamics of policymaking, where clients' needs often clashed with the competing interests of various stakeholders. As a nurse, her voice was crucial in ensuring that healthcare policy focused on clients' well-being and embraced diversity.

John's diligent work in tackling mental health concerns within the nursing community was starting to show positive outcomes. His support groups and wellness programs offered valuable spaces for nurses to discuss and address the challenges of their profession. John's work highlighted the importance of supporting those who provide care, emphasising its crucial role in the sustainability of the healthcare system in the long run. Grace furthered her expertise in elderly care through her work in geriatrics. Her approach exemplified a compassionate and successful approach to senior care, seamlessly integrating medical knowledge with a deep understanding of the unique requirements of older clients. She advocated for a healthcare system that recognised the value and worth of older people, ensuring they receive dignified and suitable care.

As the city awoke to a new day, these nurses, each in their unique manner, continued to challenge the boundaries of their profession. Their experiences went beyond being individual accounts; they formed a larger narrative about nursing in the twenty-first century. It is a tale of brilliance, advocacy, and a sincere commitment to the craft and knowledge of compassion. The future of healthcare in their hands was a promise of technological improvement and a vision of a more compassionate, egalitarian, and holistic approach to healing. Mercy Mwongozo Hospital, a beacon of knowledge in this ever-evolving environment, was a testament to their dedication. In this space, the advancement of nursing was being shaped daily.

The city was bathed in the rising sun's warm glow, casting its light upon the bustling streets below, and the day started with the usual routine of life-saving activity within the walls of Mercy Mwongozo Hospital. Every nurse, fully immersed in their responsibilities, contributed to the intricate web of compassion that set the institution apart.

Sophia encountered a new challenge upon her return from the community meeting. A young woman in a low-income neighbourhood requires immediate medical attention but, unfortunately, lacks the necessary financial resources to access the care needed. Sophia faced a challenging test of her resolve to connect healthcare with underserved communities. She collaborated with local agencies to ensure the woman received the necessary medical attention, reaffirming her belief in a healthcare system accessible to everyone, regardless of socioeconomic status.

Emma found herself in a challenging situation at the hospital's advanced wing. A client's condition had suddenly worsened, requiring prompt assessments. She relied on her expertise and intuition to make informed decisions, even with the availability of real-time data from complex monitoring systems. This scene showcased the harmonious connection between nursing and technology, a partnership where human discernment and empathy were enhanced, rather than substituted, by computers.

Meanwhile, David's telehealth session took an unexpected turn when he encountered a linguistic challenge with a distant client. This challenge underscored the importance of cultural sensitivity and effective communication in nursing. David's skill in adjusting and connecting with the client using simplified language and visual aids showcased the growing proficiency needed in contemporary nursing, going beyond clinical knowledge to encompass compassionate communication across diverse cultures.

Lina sensed her students' intense curiosity and engagement during her genomic medicine lesson. She took a moment to acknowledge their concerns, reassuring them that while medical technology continues to progress rapidly, the fundamental essence of nursing remains unchanged - the compassionate care for human life. The students found her statements thought-provoking, as they helped connect the daunting world of future technologies with the enduring principles of nursing care.

Aisha successfully resolved a cultural misunderstanding between a client and a healthcare provider as part of her community engagement program. Her adeptness in handling such challenging situations with poise and empathy resolved the immediate issue and laid the groundwork for developing more culturally sensitive healthcare protocols in the times ahead. Her work highlighted the importance of understanding and embracing different cultures and fostering empathy in nursing, recognising nurses' crucial role in a world that is becoming more interconnected and diverse.

Miriam understood the importance of engaging a wide range of individuals, including clients, technologists, and healthcare professionals, to have a more comprehensive discussion about the ethical use of AI in healthcare. He orchestrated a forum to delve into the ramifications of AI in client care, fostering a dialogue that highlighted the diverse perspectives and apprehensions surrounding healthcare technology. This endeavour demonstrated an increasing acknowledgement that the future of nursing would be shaped through collaborative efforts involving multiple stakeholders rather than in a solitary manner.

Zara's dedication to her cause earned her a seat at a roundtable discussion with policymakers, where she passionately argued for the implementation of nurse-driven initiatives in health policy. Her insights, drawn from her experiences at the bedside, offered a distinct viewpoint that often went overlooked in policymaking. Her dedication highlighted the importance of nurses' expertise in shaping policies that accurately address client needs.

Additional healthcare professionals stepped forward to share their experiences, which significantly boosted the popularity of John's mental health programs. His platform not only offered assistance but also started to reduce the negative perception associated with mental health in the workplace. The study highlighted the importance of openness and collaboration in addressing a frequently neglected aspect of mental well-being in healthcare.

Grace's day ended with a captivating conversation with one of her senior clients, who reminisced about their childhood memories. She understood that these moments of connection were as rejuvenating as the medications and therapies she provided. Her approach to senior care showcased her deep understanding of medical knowledge and her genuine appreciation for her clients' rich life experiences. It exemplified the true essence of nursing as a profession prioritising holistic care.

As darkness descended, the lights of Mercy Mwongozo Hospital continued to shine brightly, illuminating the bustling city. Within its walls, every nurse embodied the rich legacy of a profession that has consistently prioritised the well-being of humanity. Their distinct yet interconnected stories were part of a larger nursing narrative. This narrative was constantly changing while rooted in an enduring commitment to providing care and empathy and upholding the dignity of each person they attended.

CHAPTER 2

Emma's Technological Revolution

Emma's morning at Mercy Mwongozo started with a sense of anticipation. Today, she has witnessed the introduction of a cutting-edge AI-powered diagnostic system, a remarkable breakthrough in healthcare technology that holds the potential to revolutionise client care. She walked through the hospital corridors, feeling a sense of anticipation and caution about the future of medicine.

A sophisticated console awaited in the training room, its screens coming to life as the instructors commenced their demonstration. Emma was captivated as she watched the data transform into a comprehensive client profile, revealing insights beyond conventional methods' limitations. Using machine learning capabilities, the system can analyse patterns in client data and predict potential challenges before they arise.

Emma couldn't help but ponder as she delved deeper into the inner workings of the AI system: how does the nurse's role align with this emerging paradigm? Undoubtedly, the technology was impressive, but from her perspective, healthcare encompassed more than just data and algorithms. It was about understanding the individual beyond the client - their concerns, aspirations, and stories. Is it possible for a machine, regardless of its level of sophistication, to ever replicate a human carer's intuitive and empathetic abilities?

Her initial genuine challenge came earlier than anticipated. Emma depended on the AI system for insights after being assigned to a client with perplexingly unusual symptoms. As she inputted the data, the computer meticulously analysed the possibilities, suggesting a diagnosis that had eluded her. The recommendation was highly influential, leading to a treatment plan significantly improving the client's health.

Emma experienced a profound realisation due to her event. The AI system complemented her abilities and judgment rather than a substitute for them. It offered a fresh outlook on client care by blending cutting-edge technology with the expertise of healthcare professionals.

Emma's dependence on the AI system grew with each passing day, while her role as a nurse appeared to gain significance. She bridged the gap between data's precise nature and human interaction's emotional connection. Her interactions with clients, her skill in soothing their worries, and her understanding of their needs were all aspects of treatment that no technology could replicate.

Nevertheless, it could have been smoother sailing. In certain instances, the AI system's recommendations contradicted her own. These incidents were a stark reminder of the limitations of technology. Emma understood that nursing required a delicate balance between objective AI findings and the unique subjective aspects of each client's situation. The focus was on using technology as a tool rather than relying on it excessively.

Integrating artificial intelligence into her profession posed new challenges regarding client communication. Emma often had to break down intricate algorithms and data-driven decisions for clients who frequently felt overwhelmed by the vast amount of information. Her exceptional ability to communicate and educate was evident in this instance, as she effortlessly simplified complex concepts and made them relatable on a personal level.

Emma's work took on a newfound depth as she delved into AI in healthcare. The nurse's role was evolving, broadening into new areas that were once considered beyond their scope. Emma approached it with the same level of commitment and empathy that had always characterised her approach to nursing.

Mercy Mwongozo's embrace of new technology involved the implementation of advanced instruments and brought about a significant transformation in the nursing field. It gave Emma and other nurses a chance to envision their roles as healers, armed with the capabilities of technology while remaining grounded in the enduring values of empathy and compassion. Emma felt a deep sense of satisfaction and anticipation as she stepped out of the hospital that evening, the setting sun casting elongated shadows across the city. She held the destiny of nursing in her grasp, a destiny that blended the human touch with cutting-edge technology.

Emma noticed subtle shifts in the dynamics of client care as she seamlessly incorporated the AI system into her daily routine. Thanks to its remarkable capacity to process vast amounts of data, the technology brought a heightened level of accuracy to her work. However, it also raised questions about the nature of healthcare decision-making. While intuition and experience used to be prevalent, algorithms and predictive models have now emerged to offer fresh perspectives, occasionally challenging traditional methods.

Her coworkers observed this change. The implications of this new technology were often debated in the staff room. Many embraced it wholeheartedly, viewing it as a significant advancement in medicine. Others were cautious and concerned about the potential loss of the personal connection that has always been central to nursing. Emma found herself somewhere in the middle, acknowledging the potential of AI to enhance care while remaining steadfast in her belief that human connection was essential in nursing.

A challenging case crossed her path one afternoon—an elderly and feeble client presented with symptoms that were challenging to interpret. The AI system provided a diagnosis, but the client's demeanour hinted at a deeper narrative. Emma dedicated her time to the client, attentively listening to his life story, anxieties, and fears. Emma gained valuable insights not previously documented through this conversation, leading her to adjust the treatment plan. The client's condition improved not only due to the technology but also because of the care and attention she provided.

This event solidified Emma's understanding of her position in this new era of nursing. She possessed a deep understanding and analysis of technology, going beyond mere usage. Her remarkable skill in integrating the AI system's data with her clinical expertise and understanding her clients' needs was invaluable. She acted as a connection between the realms of statistics and the human experience.

This groundbreaking advancement had a far-reaching impact that extended beyond the confines of the hospital. Emma actively participated in community outreach programs, educating the public about the advantages and constraints of cutting-edge healthcare technologies. Her goal was to educate and provide comfort, showcasing that even with advanced technology and intricate algorithms, the fundamental objective of healthcare remained unchanged: to provide compassionate and effective treatment.

Emma's foray into AI in healthcare went beyond being a mere professional test; it was also a personal odyssey of self-development. She acquired fresh skills, learned to pose novel inquiries, and gained a new outlook on her job. Technology has brought forth previously unimaginable opportunities while also emphasising the timeless ideals of nursing. Navigating the delicate balance between innovation and tradition, between the digital and the human, required careful consideration.

Emma pondered her journeys as she departed the hospital one evening, with the city lights gradually illuminating her surroundings. She was at the forefront of the evolving healthcare industry, transforming the way. With each step, she carried the rich legacy of nursing - a tradition rooted in empathy, kindness, and meaningful relationships, now amplified by the potential of technology. The future of healthcare rested in her capable hands and the hands of nurses like her - a future filled with promise and challenges, a mix of excitement and apprehension. As Emma journeyed, she stumbled upon a novel approach to hone her craft, bringing a renewed sense of meaning and satisfaction to her beloved work.

Emma's tenure at Mercy Mwongozo developed alongside a broader transformation in the nursing field. With the increasing integration of technology into healthcare, nurses found themselves at the intersection of human empathy and technical innovation. This combination of skills was increasingly essential, no longer just a valuable asset.

Emma's daily routine now encompassed more than just her nursing duties. The tasks involved analysing data from the AI system, collaborating with IT teams to enhance algorithms, and keeping abreast of the latest advancements in healthcare technologies. She assumed the role of a mediator between clients and the increasingly prevalent technical instruments used in their care.

Emma strongly supported integrating technology that enhanced, rather than detracted from, the nurse-client interaction during discussions with the hospital's administrative and technology departments. She highlighted the significance of user-friendly technologies enabling nurses to prioritise client care instead of grappling with complex software. She advocated for the involvement of clinical workers in the design and deployment of new technology, ensuring that it prioritised the needs of people at the bedside.

There were a multitude of challenges. Maintaining client data's privacy and security in an ever-growing digital landscape is a significant concern. Emma actively sought educational opportunities to deepen her understanding of the importance of cybersecurity in the healthcare industry. She shared this information with her staff, ensuring everyone was well-informed about the highest data management standards and client confidentiality.

One challenge that arose was the emotional aspect of nursing in a highly advanced environment. Although the AI system proved highly beneficial in diagnosing and treating clients, it fell short of replacing the essential human qualities of compassion and comfort crucial in nursing. Emma discovered she dedicated much time to her clients, offering them comfort and attentive support. She skillfully combined the effectiveness of technology with the compassion of individualised attention.

This new era also brought fresh possibilities for client education and engagement innovation. Emma utilised digital tools to enhance the accessibility of information regarding her clients' conditions and medical interventions. She found that clients with a deeper understanding were more engaged in their care, improving outcomes. Through technology, clients could access education and gain empowerment, transforming it from an obstacle to a tool.

Emma's journey in nursing and technology was a collaborative effort. She was part of a collective of healthcare experts delving into this uncharted territory. They exchanged their insights, gained knowledge from each other, and collaboratively adapted to the changing healthcare landscape. This group, which extended beyond Mercy Mwongozo's doors, consisted of specialists from various fields, each contributing their distinct perspectives to the discussion.

The responsibilities of nurses in healthcare technology research and development have also grown. Emma actively contributed to test initiatives, offering valuable feedback and innovative ideas that played a crucial role in shaping client-centric solutions. Her deep understanding of client care was critical to identifying new tools' practical uses and potential risks.

With the advancement of technology, the ethical dilemmas it brought along also evolved. Emma actively engaged in discussions and forums regarding the impact of artificial intelligence on healthcare decision-making. These discussions were crucial in establishing policies and procedures that promoted the responsible and ethical use of technology in client care.

Her experiences highlighted the importance of continuous learning in the field of nursing. Emma was committed to constantly expanding her knowledge to keep pace with the ever-evolving world of technology. She made it a point to participate in workshops, seminars, and online courses. Her colleagues embraced a solid dedication to knowledge, cultivating an environment of progress and creativity at Mercy Mwongozo.

Despite the rapid progress of technology, some aspects of nursing have remained unchanged: the demanding schedules, the rollercoaster of emotions, the joy of witnessing a client's recovery, and the sorrow of losing them. These experiences, passed down by nurses for generations, have remained the profession's bedrock.

Emma witnessed Mercy Mwongozo's remarkable transformation into a cutting-edge hospital centre over several years. However, its workers' unwavering dedication and compassion defined the hospital's identity. The hospital's lights illuminated the night sky, symbolising hope and compassion and guiding those in need.

Emma's story showcased the ability of nurses to adapt and persevere amid change. She epitomised the advancement of nursing, a profession that not only embraced the digital age but also played a crucial role in shaping it. Her approach combined the best of both worlds - blending traditional methods with cutting-edge innovation, balancing empathy and analytical thinking, and seamlessly integrating personal interaction with the precision of computer technology.

Upon deep contemplation of her journey, Emma realised that the transformation in healthcare lay not solely in technology advancements but in its application to enhance clients' well-being. The focus was on utilising every available resource, whether digital or otherwise, to provide the highest quality of care. At the heart of it all was the nurse, a steadfast presence in the ever-evolving world of healthcare, maintaining the delicate equilibrium between compassionate care and technological advancements.

Emma and other nurses were not just carers in this new era; they were trailblazers, leading the charge in a world where technology and compassion intertwine. They created a groundbreaking form of healthcare that prioritised precision, effectiveness, and empathy. As the world evolved, they continued to lead the way in the healthcare profession, adjusting, acquiring knowledge, and showing compassion.

Emma's interaction with her clients expanded as technology progressed. Through her interactions with AI systems, she gained a deeper appreciation for the human aspects of nursing. Each client encounter was a reminder that every information set had a story, a life, and an individual seeking medical attention, compassion, and empathy.

The hospital environment started to embody the harmonious blend of advanced technology and compassionate care. Screens and monitors hummed in harmony with the calming voices of nurses engaging in gentle conversations with their clients. Mercy Mwongozo's impressive fusion of technology and client care captivated Emma and her colleagues. Emma was often at the forefront of these excursions, passionately showcasing the advancements and elucidating their practical implications in nursing. These contacts highlighted the hospital's standing as a frontrunner in healthcare innovation while equipping Emma and her team with insights into global healthcare trends.

Technology has significantly influenced client follow-ups and remote care. Emma utilised telehealth systems to communicate with clients after discharge, ensuring a seamless continuation of care. This approach enhanced client outcomes and provided a more comprehensive understanding of their recovery journey, connecting the dots between hospital and home care.

The journey, though, was not without its challenges. The rapid pace of technological advancement could be overwhelming at times, prompting Emma to emphasise the importance of self-care to herself and her team. She stressed the importance of maintaining a healthy work-life balance, highlighting how crucial it was for nurses to prioritise their well-being to provide high-quality care.

Emma's role in this evolving healthcare environment went beyond the confines of the hospital. She developed a keen interest in community activities, advocating for improved health literacy and increased technological access in marginalised communities. She dedicated herself to reducing health disparities and ensuring that advancements in healthcare technology were accessible to all.

Emma's insights were highly valued in team meetings and planning sessions. Her extensive clinical experience and understanding of technology made her a valuable asset in shaping the hospital's long-term strategies. She was crucial in advancing client-centred care models that integrated technology while prioritising each client's needs.

Emma's approach to nursing education developed in tandem with the progress of technology. She dedicated herself to curriculum creation, ensuring that nursing students were well-equipped to excel in a healthcare setting enhanced by technology. Her valuable contributions have played a crucial role in shaping a new generation of nurses who possess the necessary skills and knowledge to navigate the challenges and possibilities of contemporary healthcare.

Emma remained committed to the core principles of nursing throughout her journey. She understood the importance of recognising technology as a tool rather than a replacement for the human element of care. Her unique and conventional approach to nursing became a model for others.

Emma's work had a profound influence that extended far beyond the confines of Mercy Mwongozo. She emerged as a prominent figure in the broader healthcare community, advocating for policies and practices that promoted technology integration in client care while emphasising the importance of the human touch. Her insights and unique experiences added depth to the ongoing conversation surrounding the future of nursing, a future that brimmed with vitality, challenges, and potential.

Emma envisioned boundless opportunities as she gazed towards the future. She was at the forefront of the ever-evolving healthcare landscape. However, one thing remained unwavering: her unwavering commitment to providing compassionate, client-centred care. Emma and her colleagues' nurses served as a poignant reminder of the enduring significance of human connection in the healing process, even as technology revolutionised every aspect of our lives. They bridged the gap between cutting-edge medicine and the timeless practice of compassion, paving the way for a harmonious future where both could thrive.

CHAPTER 3

The Call of David

A midst the global health crisis that swept continents, profoundly reshaping the healthcare landscape, David's journey at Mercy Mwongozo took a significant shift. Amidst this period of turmoil, he stumbled upon his true passion, a revelation that would revolutionise his career and his perspective on nursing.

The hospital corridors, typically filled with daily medical care routines, became the battleground for a fight against an invisible adversary. Much like his colleagues, David found himself thrust into the heart of the crisis, facing unprecedented challenges in his work. Each day, he presented new challenges, each more complex than the last, pushing his skills and determination to their limits.

When confronted with this daunting obstacle, David tapped into a profound reservoir of inner fortitude. He dedicated himself to his work, caring for those affected by viruses, comforting those in distress, and supporting families facing illness and uncertainty. The crisis was not just a medical challenge; it served as a testament to the strength of the human spirit, and David demonstrated his empathy and determination in confronting it.

David's engagement developed as the situation unfolded. He discovered himself by clients' bedsides and at the forefront of public health activities. He actively engaged in community outreach, educating individuals about the virus, methods of prevention, and the importance of vaccination. His nursing skills were enhanced by a recently discovered knack for communication and public involvement.

The global scale of the crisis opened David's eyes to the intricate links between health and society. He observed the impact of public health policies on individuals' lives and how socioeconomic factors influenced health outcomes. This realisation redirected his career towards a broader perspective on global health, moving away from the direct care of individual clients.

David's experiences during the crisis highlighted the importance of collaboration in the healthcare field. He worked closely with doctors, epidemiologists, and other healthcare professionals, bringing their expertise to the battle against the virus. David was deeply impressed by this multidisciplinary approach, highlighting the significance of considering various perspectives when tackling complex health issues.

The crisis also presented chances for self-reflection. David pondered the profound meaning of his profession during the late-night hours following extended shifts. Nursing became more than a job to him; it was a deep commitment to supporting humanity in its most fragile moments. The crisis had not only challenged his abilities; it had also deepened his understanding of the complexities of human existence.

Fueled by these encounters, David envisioned a future where his efforts could wield a more significant impact. He started engaging with policymakers, offering his expertise and insights to contribute to developing health policies influenced by real-life experiences on the front. His ideas, forged amid a crisis, were crucial in formulating strategies to enhance the healthcare system.

David's encounter with the global health crisis profoundly impacted him. He rose to prominence as a nurse and a staunch advocate for public health, a respected figure in the community, and a catalyst for transforming healthcare. The crisis had completely shifted his career aspirations, leading him towards a path where he could make a more significant difference.

As the world slowly emerged from the crisis, David carried the knowledge he had gained and the experiences of those challenging times with him. The event changed him and solidified his dedication to nursing, a remarkable and demanding profession. After the crisis, David envisioned a future where he could apply his insights to improve the well-being of communities and societies at large rather than focusing solely on individuals.

His story showcased nurses' unwavering determination and flexibility, highlighting their crucial role in shaping the future of healthcare despite challenging circumstances. David's unique insight led him to a fresh outlook on his job, which was expansive, all-encompassing, and intricately intertwined with the world around him. Through his journey, he unearthed more than just a job but a profound sense of purpose that reached far beyond the confines of Mercy Mwongozo and connected with the broader, worldwide story of well-being and restoration.

David's position at Mercy Mwongozo and in the broader community developed as society adapted to the changed circumstances after the crisis. His experiences during the global health crisis instilled in him a strong sense of responsibility towards public health. He grew more engaged in initiatives to prevent such outbreaks, advocating for more robust healthcare systems well-equipped to handle such situations.

David's interactions with individuals most affected by the crisis left a lasting impression on him. He realised that healthcare encompassed more than just the treatment of diseases. It involved a deep understanding of the socioeconomic factors influencing one's health. He observed healthcare access and outcomes disparities, which fueled his dedication to achieving health equity. He embarked on community initiatives to improve healthcare accessibility, especially in marginalised areas.

He actively participated in global health conferences, advocating for frontline nurses' perspectives. David shared his insights on the pandemic response, highlighting the importance of forward-thinking and international collaboration in addressing health crises. He stressed the importance of nurses in public health policy and decision-making, not just as carers.

David took on the role of a mentor at Mercy Mwongozo, offering his valuable insights and helping younger nurses navigate the complexities of modern healthcare. He encouraged them to expand their thinking beyond the boundaries of the hospital and consider the broader implications of their work. He fostered an environment of constant learning and adaptability, which proved crucial in navigating the rapidly evolving healthcare industry.

David has collaborated with educational institutions to help develop global health and public health policy curricula. He was determined to ensure that the upcoming generation of nurses was well-equipped to tackle global health issues. His lectures encompassed a wide range of topics, including clinical skills and the ethical responsibilities of nursing from an international standpoint.

David's understanding of the emotional and mental health aspects of nursing had also expanded due to the crisis. He had witnessed the profound effects of the crisis on healthcare personnel and advocated for increased mental health support within the healthcare sector. Through his dedication, he successfully implemented wellness programs at Mercy Mwongozo, providing nurses and other healthcare staff with the necessary tools to manage the challenges of their profession.

David found a renewed sense of direction on his journey. The global health crisis compelled him to expand his perspective and venture into new possibilities in nursing. He had embraced roles as an advocate, mentor, and leader, demonstrating the same unwavering dedication and empathy he had shown as a nurse.

David's account highlighted the evolving responsibilities of nurses in the modern era. They had transcended the confines of traditional hospital duties and became indispensable contributors to shaping healthcare policies, imparting knowledge to future generations, and addressing worldwide health challenges. David's journey exemplified the diverse and ever-evolving nature of the nursing field.

David was optimistic about his prospects for the future. He recognised challenges yet also recognised the immense potential for nurses to impact healthcare profoundly. Through his journey, he discovered that nursing had a greater purpose beyond just a profession. It catalysed transformation, enhancing the well-being of individuals and communities. David, a nurse, was at the forefront of navigating the dynamic landscape of healthcare, equipped with extensive expertise, profound understanding, and a sincere dedication to the well-being of people.

David's fresh outlook on nursing and global health inspired him to pursue initiatives beyond conventional healthcare boundaries. He spearheaded initiatives that tackled immediate health concerns and focused on proactive measures, recognising that comprehensive healthcare involves nurturing overall well-being.

One such endeavour was a community outreach program focused on school health education. David was convinced that providing early education on health, hygiene, and nutrition could have a profound effect on future generations. He collaborated with teachers and health educators to develop engaging programs for children and informative for their families. This approach aimed to build a strong understanding of health early on, fostering a community better equipped to handle health challenges.

David expanded his interests to include global health studies alongside his community activities. He dedicated himself to researching illness patterns, vaccine efficacy, and the long-term consequences of the recent global health crisis. His deep understanding of the subject enhanced these investigations, connecting academic research with real-world applications. This study not only benefited the scholarly community but also had a significant impact on public health policies and practices.

David had a deep understanding of the importance of mental health, both for his clients and his colleagues. The global financial crisis has dramatically impacted the well-being of individuals worldwide. He initiated support groups for healthcare professionals, providing them a platform to exchange their experiences and coping mechanisms. He ensured that the well-being of his clients included comprehensive mental health care in their treatment programs. He advocated for a holistic health approach that emphasised physical and emotional well-being.

David's expertise and extensive background at Mercy Mwongozo profoundly impacted the hospital's approach to anticipating and addressing health crises. He worked closely with the management to develop effective disaster response strategies, enhancing the hospital's readiness for future emergencies. His primary focus was on constructing a system that was adaptable, effective, and centred around the client's needs.

David consistently demonstrated a high level of care and expertise in client interactions. He quickly recognised that every client encounter presented a chance to educate and inspire. He dedicated himself to his clients, educating them about preventive health practices and encouraging them to participate actively in their well-being. These conversations often went beyond the professional setting, as he engaged with clients and their families, building trust and empathy.

David's efforts extended to a global scale as well. He attended international health conferences on Mercy Mwongozo's behalf, exchanging knowledge with experts worldwide. These forums offered a platform for exchanging knowledge and connecting with like-minded individuals who could collaborate on tackling global health issues. David understood the international nature of health challenges and the need for a comprehensive approach.

He also incorporated policy advocacy into his nursing perspective. David guided legislators on healthcare workforce demands, client care standards, and public health measures. He believed nurses should significantly impact shaping health policies due to their firsthand experience caring for clients. His efforts aimed to elevate the nursing profession, emphasising the importance of nurses as essential members of the healthcare system rather than just carers.

David's journey also encompassed personal growth. He pursued further education, expanding his public health and healthcare management knowledge. His commitment to continuous learning allowed him to stay current on healthcare trends and apply this knowledge to his responsibilities. He embraced a lifelong pursuit of knowledge, passionately championing his beliefs and guiding others, roles he never anticipated when he first entered nursing.

David frequently pondered the trajectory of his career during moments of deep reflection. Throughout his nursing career, he has encountered numerous obstacles, acquired knowledge, and experienced great satisfaction, from direct client care to community involvement to international endeavours. He had witnessed the power of nursing to heal, educate, advocate, and lead. His encounters during the global health crisis ignited a profound change in his profession and his perspective on life and healthcare.

David was brimming with confidence and determination as he gazed into the future. The healthcare industry has always been in a state of constant evolution, presenting a multitude of challenges and opportunities. However, it was clear that individuals with a deep understanding and expertise would play a crucial role in addressing these challenges, and nurses like him were no exception. They would excel as advocates for clients, educators for the next generation, experts in health policy, and pioneers in pushing the boundaries of medical science.

David's narrative showcased the expanding influence of nurses in the modern era, reaching far beyond the confines of hospitals and into the realms of public health, policy, and global health. His journey mirrored the dynamic nature of nursing, a field constantly developing, expanding, and impacting individuals' lives. David exemplified the nursing spirit, showing deep compassion, unwavering resilience, and a solid determination to make a meaningful impact in healthcare.

David's influence at Mercy Mwongozo Hospital reverberated throughout the entire healthcare system. He gained recognition for his expertise in combining various disciplines and fostering partnerships that enhanced the quality of client care. His goal was to create a healthcare model that seamlessly integrated the expertise of multiple professions, guaranteeing a comprehensive approach to treatment and recovery.

His passion for this idea drove him to collaborate closely with the hospital's IT department to seamlessly incorporate data analytics into client care. This program seeks to enhance diagnostic precision, tailor treatment methods, and predict client outcomes with greater precision. David's input was invaluable to this project as he provided the clinical perspective, ensuring the technology was designed with the client's needs in mind.

David's community health programs started to yield positive results beyond the confines of the hospital. His school programs produced impressive outcomes, fostering greater health awareness among children and their families. He viewed this as a crucial measure in promoting a culture prioritising health consciousness, where the emphasis on prevention was just as significant as treatment.

David recognised the worldwide nature of healthcare and understood the importance of cultural competence in nursing. He strongly supported having a diverse nursing workforce, recognising the value of different perspectives and experiences in delivering culturally sensitive care. He developed cultural sensitivity training programs at Mercy Mwongozo to enhance client-nurse relationships and improve outcomes.

David successfully balanced his various roles while still prioritising his connection with clients. He passionately believed that providing direct client care was the core of nursing, and it helped him stay connected to his work. These contacts served as a powerful reminder of the profound impact nursing can have on individuals' lives. Every client story reinforced his determination to create a healthcare system that prioritises clients and is easily accessible to all.

David inspired and guided a new generation of nurses as a mentor. He imparted his wisdom and insights to them, instilling in them a broader perspective of nursing that went beyond conventional duties. He encouraged them to approach situations with a thoughtful mindset, to be flexible, and to prioritise the client's well-being consistently. His guidance extended beyond the technical aspects, offering support to students as they navigated the intricacies of the healthcare system and the challenges of the nursing profession.

David's path was filled with challenges. Juggling his multitude of tasks often required significant effort and time. Nevertheless, his passion for nursing and public health propelled him forward. He received motivation and backing from his colleagues and loved ones, who embraced his vision and provided unwavering support throughout his journey.

David's work profoundly influenced the hospital and the broader healthcare community. He emerged as a catalyst for change, advocating for policies that improved clients' and healthcare staff's health and well-being. His contributions were acknowledged on various platforms, highlighting the crucial role of nurses in transforming healthcare.

David became aware of the significant growth he had experienced in his professional and personal life as he contemplated his journey. His journey in nursing was a remarkable, challenging, and fulfilling experience. He has observed the profession evolve as it responds to new challenges and possibilities. Through his experiences, he had come to appreciate the importance of perseverance, understanding, and continuous growth.

David was brimming with optimism as he gazed into the future. He envisioned a future where healthcare would be more inclusive, proactive, and focused on the client's needs. He envisioned a world where nurses were crucial in shaping health policy, education, and innovation. His experience showcased the profound influence of nursing on healthcare and society in the long run.

David's narrative captured the profound evolution of the nursing profession, encompassing more than just his personal experiences. It was a journey of growth, overcoming challenges, and expanding horizons. David and other nurses were at the forefront, showcasing that nursing encompassed more than just caregiving. It involved changing lives, influencing policies, and propelling healthcare towards an equal future.

CHAPTER 4

Lina's Classroom of the Future

L ina was at the forefront of a subtle revolution in nursing education. A new era was dawning within the confines of her classroom at Mercy Mwongozo's training centre, where traditional methods were being questioned and reshaped. Her goal was clear: she aimed to educate nurses with technical expertise and the ability to think critically, develop new ideas, and take charge in the healthcare industry.

Gone were the days of mindlessly memorising and passively absorbing information. Lina's classroom buzzed with animated discussions, in-depth analyses, and collaborative problem-solving sessions. She promoted a practical approach to learning, where students were encouraged to inquire, explore, and apply their knowledge in real-life situations. The classroom was a vibrant and stimulating environment, a crucible of knowledge where aspiring nurses were moulded.

Lina's educational model was highly focused on utilising technology. She integrated state-of-the-art digital resources, such as simulations and virtual reality, into her classroom instruction to provide students with a lifelike experience of clinical scenarios. This approach not only enhanced their knowledge but also equipped them for the ever-evolving advancements in healthcare technology.

Lina's educational innovation, however, extended beyond technology. She highlighted the importance of developing soft skills, including effective communication, empathy, and ethical decisions. Her curriculum showcased a comprehensive understanding of the challenges in contemporary healthcare, encompassing classes on cultural competency, mental health, and client advocacy. She acknowledged the complexity of the nursing profession and the diverse range of skills it demands.

Her students, who came from various backgrounds and had unique perspectives, enriched the classroom. Lina saw the value in embracing diversity, recognising its potential to enhance education and prepare nurses for multicultural environments. She fostered an environment where all students' perspectives were highly regarded, and every encounter was seen as a chance for growth.

Lina also invited healthcare professionals from diverse sectors to impart their knowledge and share their experiences with her students. These guest lectures and workshops gave students valuable perspectives on the interdisciplinary nature of healthcare and emphasised the significance of collaboration and teamwork.

Lina's teaching methods had a profound influence that extended far beyond the confines of the classroom. Her students were recognised for their sharp analytical skills, adaptability, and eagerness to tackle the challenges of contemporary nursing. They were thoughtful advocates, adept at manoeuvring through the complexities of healthcare systems and guiding others with empathy and expertise.

Lina encountered numerous challenges in her pursuit of nursing education. She often found herself at odds with those who held more traditional views and were sceptical of her methods. But she continued, driven by her conviction that nursing education must adapt to meet the changing needs of healthcare.

Her accomplishments started gaining recognition not just within Mercy Mwongozo but also among the wider nursing education community. Lina was invited to conferences and seminars to share her expertise and perspectives. Her idea sparked lively debate and thoughtful discussion, pushing educators to reevaluate their methods and embrace new ideas.

Lina experienced a profound feeling of satisfaction as she contemplated her journey. She equipped her students with the essential skills and inspired them to approach things from a fresh perspective, embrace bravery, and challenge conventional limits. She had nurtured a new generation of nurses who possessed a strong sense of self-assurance and a burning desire to revolutionise the future of healthcare.

Lina was brimming with enthusiasm as she prepared for another day in her classroom the next day. She played a pivotal role in shaping the future of the ever-changing healthcare industry. She recognised the potential of her students to shape the future of nursing, envisioning a future filled with creativity, diversity, and optimism. Her classroom was a transformative space where future nurses were empowered to become healthcare leaders, equipped with the knowledge and skills they had honed under her guidance.

Lina's innovative teaching methods have significantly impacted the Mercy Mwongozo community, leaving a lasting impression on her students and fellow educators. She became a catalyst for change, motivating others to explore innovative approaches to education. The transformation was slow but unmistakable. Classrooms throughout the training centre were filled with vibrant discussions, collaborative learning, and a curious atmosphere.

Lina's focus on client-centred treatment was one of her most notable accomplishments. She instilled in her students the importance of recognising the distinctiveness of each client and understanding their personal stories, challenges, and needs. Her students were encouraged to go beyond the surface and connect with clients on a deeper level—this strategy aimed to revolutionise the connection between nurse and client, fostering trust and comprehension.

Lina conducted research alongside her teaching to evaluate the effectiveness of her methods. She diligently collected data, meticulously analysed the results, and confidently shared her well-founded conclusions. Her research showcased the efficacy of her nursing education approach, which enhanced learning outcomes and improved client care. This evidence strengthened her argument for reforming nursing education.

Lina's objective also encompassed the pursuit of continuous education for registered nurses. She developed workshops and training programs to assist individuals in keeping pace with the fast-paced developments in healthcare, ensuring their skills and expertise remained current. These programs were highly regarded, with nurses from Mercy Mwongozo and other hospitals enthusiastically participating.

She demonstrated a deep commitment to education that extended far beyond the confines of the hospital. Lina actively engaged with the community by organising health fairs and public awareness campaigns. She brought her students along, providing them with practical experience and a chance to put their knowledge into practice. These outreach programs positively impacted the community's and students' understanding of public health matters.

Lina's profile grew, opening up new opportunities for collaboration. She worked closely with technology businesses to develop innovative learning tools, partnered with healthcare organisations to enhance care models, and engaged with lawmakers to advocate for advancements in nursing education. Her connections expanded, creating a network of collaboration that enhanced her impact in the nursing field.

Lina found great satisfaction in the accomplishments of her students in their respective careers, which was the most fulfilling aspect of her journey. They were recognised for their sharp analytical skills, empathetic approach, and ability to guide others in diverse healthcare environments. They emerged as advocates for clients, pioneers of new ideas, and influential figures in their communities.

Lina often reflected on the journey she had embarked upon. It had been challenging, but every hurdle had only strengthened her determination. She had observed a change in nursing education that she had helped to cultivate. The realisation of her vision for a future school was evident in the high quality of nurses entering the sector.

Lina was optimistic about the future. She envisioned a world where nursing education constantly evolves, embracing the latest technology, approaches, and ideologies. She observed a society where nurses were not only carers but also pioneers, trailblazers, and catalysts for change. Her diligent work has laid the foundation for what lies ahead, and she eagerly anticipates witnessing the progress that the upcoming generation of nurses will make.

Lina's classroom of the future was a perpetual journey of learning, an eternal quest for knowledge, and an unwavering commitment to client care. It was a hub of knowledge and innovation, where the future of nursing was being moulded through classes and the brilliance of its students. Lina found immense satisfaction in her career and the delight of making a lasting impact on the healthcare industry throughout her journey.

Lina's classroom became a hub of innovation and motivation, a space where the nursing profession's future was actively moulded. Her work started to make a significant impact beyond her students' immediate sphere of influence. Graduates of the program, now employed in various healthcare settings, often came back to discuss their experiences, creating diverse learning opportunities and practical applications.

Lina's teaching methods started to influence the nursing curriculum significantly. Focusing on technical proficiency and holistic care, her approach became a role model for nursing programs seeking to update their teaching methods. She was often sought after to speak at educational forums and conferences, where she generously shared her vast knowledge and valuable experiences with a broader audience of educators and healthcare professionals.

Lina's focus on fostering critical thinking and problem-solving skills aimed to empower her students to become catalysts for change within the healthcare system, going beyond the role of mere nurses. She encouraged them to question established protocols and practices and to always strive for ways to enhance client care. This approach motivated numerous students to actively engage in quality improvement projects within their respective hospital settings, leading to the emergence of innovative ideas from the ground up.

The dynamic nature of the healthcare industry drove her focus on continuous learning and flexibility. Lina acknowledged the challenges nurses encounter today, understanding that the future will introduce new demands and expectations. She emphasised the importance of informing her students about the latest medical developments, public health trends, and healthcare technology advancements.

Lina's educational approach incorporated the utilisation of technology not only for instruction but also for connecting her students with the worldwide nursing community. Engaging in virtual exchanges with nursing students and professionals worldwide became a regular part of her curriculum. Through these exchanges, her students gained a deeper understanding of global health issues, cultural diversity in healthcare, and the universal challenges and triumphs of nursing.

Lina also highlighted the importance of transdisciplinary learning. She collaborated with various departments at Mercy Mwongozo and other institutions to coordinate lectures and workshops. Through her multidisciplinary approach, she helped her pupils develop a deeper comprehension of healthcare, emphasising the interconnectedness of various medical and allied health professions.

She was deeply committed to furthering nursing education and researched the field. Lina was the primary catalyst behind studies that explored the outcomes of her groundbreaking teaching methods. Her research showcased the effectiveness of interactive, technology-enhanced, and student-centred learning in nursing education. These findings have significantly impacted the scholarly discourse on nursing education, shaping the perspectives of educators and policymakers alike.

The success of Lina's pupils in clinical settings is a testament to the effectiveness of her teaching methods. They were often commended for their clinical skills, analytical thinking, and readiness for leadership roles. Lina was filled with immense joy at their achievement, which affirmed the value of her life's work.

Lina faced numerous challenges along her journey. Resistance to change is a common theme in various fields, and nursing education is no different. Convincing those resistant to new ideas requires patience, commitment, and tangible outcomes. The outcomes achieved by her students, along with the increasing body of research supporting her methods, gradually alleviated much of the initial resistance.

Lina's dedication and hard work had a profound impact not only on the success of her students but also on the transformation of nursing education. She initiated a movement that emphasised innovation, fostered critical thinking, and prioritised comprehensive client care.

Lina was deeply committed to pushing the boundaries of nursing education as she eagerly anticipated what lay ahead. She observed a society where nurses fulfilled caregiving roles and took on leadership, education, and advocacy responsibilities for their clients and communities. She envisioned a nursing profession that was adaptable and well-equipped to navigate the challenges of a constantly evolving healthcare industry.

Lina laid the foundation for this upcoming development in her forthcoming classroom. She motivated a new generation of nurses to think critically, challenge conventional thinking, and pursue excellence in every aspect of their profession. Her impact on the nursing profession was profound, and her legacy will endure in the hearts and minds of her students, who will uphold the values of innovation and compassion in healthcare.

Lina's influence on the future of nursing education reached far beyond the Mercy Mwongozo campus. Her methods sparked a nationwide network of educators, leading to a collaborative exchange of ideas and best practices. This network was crucial in promoting a more dynamic and responsive nursing curriculum nationwide, bringing about significant changes.

Lina consistently sought feedback from her students to foster ongoing development. She regarded them not merely as students but as valuable contributors to the educational process. This continuous feedback loop enabled her to consistently enhance and broaden her teaching methods, ensuring their relevance and efficacy.

Her classroom was a hub for experimenting with innovative teaching methods. Lina incorporated the latest technological advancements into her training, ranging from cutting-edge client simulation systems to state-of-the-art diagnostic tools driven by artificial intelligence. These tools enhanced her students' learning experience and equipped them for the advanced world of modern healthcare.

Lina recognised the importance of emotional intelligence in nursing. She implemented courses that emphasised the cultivation of empathy, stress management, and resilience - all essential skills in healthcare. Her approach focused on the emotional and psychological aspects of nursing, equipping her students to handle the profession's challenges with empathy and composure.

Lina's educational perspective was enriched by her students' achievements in leadership positions within and outside clinical settings. Several of her past students have progressed to become leaders in nursing teams, have impacted legislation, and have made advancements in client care. Their achievements showcased the success of Lina's instructional methods.

Lina started publishing her work to disseminate her thoughts and experiences on a larger platform. Her nursing education essays and publications garnered attention in academic circles, sparking lively discussions and inspiring other educators to adopt similar methodologies.

She had a broad perspective on global health education. Lina fostered partnerships with nursing schools across the globe, creating exchange programs that offered students valuable insights into healthcare from an international standpoint. These events expanded the students' outlook and fostered a worldwide camaraderie among nurses.

Lina's unwavering dedication to nursing education innovation was paralleled by her intense focus on her students' personal and professional growth. She became a guiding light for many others, offering support in their professional endeavours and inspiring them to chase after their aspirations. She had unwavering confidence in her students' capabilities and consistently went the extra mile to provide them with opportunities to succeed.

Lina's work in nursing education profoundly impacted the nurses she trained. They became highly skilled in their clinical abilities and developed a strong capacity for adaptability, empathy, and resilience in the face of a rapidly evolving healthcare landscape. Her students were a testament to her unwavering commitment to nursing education, each one embodying her passion for academic excellence.

Lina experienced profound satisfaction as she surveyed her classroom, brimming with enthusiastic and engaged children. She had closely observed and actively contributed to the progress of nursing education. Her journey showcased the impact of ingenuity, commitment, and passion in shaping a career trajectory.

Her narrative went beyond that of a typical educator; it encapsulated the journey of a forward-thinking individual who revolutionised the concept of nursing education. Lina had planted the seeds for a promising future in healthcare in her visionary classroom, where nurses were empowered, clients received compassionate care, and education was constantly evolving. Lina's unwavering dedication and passion have been a guiding light for aspiring nurses, leaving a lasting impact on the profession.

CHAPTER 5

Aisha's Diverse Story

Aisha's tenure at Mercy Mwongozo was marked by her unwavering commitment to fostering diversity and creating an inclusive environment. With her extensive experience as a nurse, she has witnessed firsthand the profound influence that ethnic diversity can have on client care and the overall dynamics within a hospital. Her narrative went beyond the challenge of diversity and focused on fostering an inclusive environment where all voices were acknowledged and all cultures were respected.

Aisha noticed a recurring pattern in Mercy Mwongozo's hallways that troubled her. Aisha's impact on diversity and inclusion extended beyond the confines of Mercy Mwongozo Hospital. Her endeavours captured the interest of the broader healthcare community, setting a precedent for hospitals to address diversity in a substantial and noteworthy manner.

Mercy Mwongozo's modifications sparked a broader conversation within the healthcare industry. Aisha has been invited to speak at conferences and symposiums, where she has enthusiastically shared her experiences and techniques for developing a diverse workforce. Her presentations blended personal anecdotes, pragmatic solutions, and a passionate plea, motivating other organisations to seek increased diversity.

Aisha's dedication to promoting diversity became evident in various aspects of client care at Mercy Mwongozo. The team's diverse composition fostered a heightened understanding and empathy toward clients' cultural concerns. Language barriers were minimised, cultural misunderstandings were addressed, and client satisfaction levels improved. The hospital started to embody a true reflection of the community it served.

Aisha played a significant role in developing a curriculum that promotes inclusivity in the hospital's training programs. She utilised case studies and scenarios emphasising different cultural contexts, ensuring that new nurses were better equipped to navigate the intricacies of diverse backgrounds. This curriculum modification aimed to go beyond imparting knowledge, seeking to mould attitudes and foster empathy among future healthcare practitioners.

She had a strong passion for promoting diversity and inclusiveness, which she also applied to client education. Aisha played a crucial role in developing client education materials in multiple languages and formats, guaranteeing that every client, regardless of language or cultural background, could easily understand and benefit from valuable health information.

Nevertheless, Aisha's work had a profound impact on the lives of her colleagues. Professionals from diverse backgrounds started to feel greater recognition and belonging, leading to a heightened commitment to their work. A diverse range of perspectives was welcomed and frequently valued in the professional environment.

The journey was filled with its fair share of challenges. Aisha faced resistance and doubt along the way, but her unwavering commitment and resolve remained steadfast. She understood that change necessitates patience and tireless dedication, particularly when reshaping deeply rooted concepts and habits.

Aisha's vision of a diverse and inclusive healthcare environment gradually came to fruition at Mercy Mwongozo. The hospital had transformed into a compassionate community that mirrored the diverse tapestry of the society it catered to. Clients and staff alike experienced a strong sense of community, highlighting the significance of inclusivity in cultivating a more empathetic and prosperous healthcare system.

Aisha experienced a profound sense of fulfilment as she pondered her journey. She had not only addressed the issue of diversity in her institution but also played a crucial role in its transformation. Her story served as a source of motivation for individuals in the healthcare field and anyone seeking to create a positive impact in their community.

Aisha's account of diversity at Mercy Mwongozo was a powerful reminder of the essential role of embracing diversity in ensuring that an institution can deliver top-notch care. Her impact will endure, serving as a source of inspiration and guidance for generations of healthcare professionals. She exemplified the core values of inclusivity, understanding, and respect in healthcare.

Aisha's contributions at Mercy Mwongozo Hospital shone brightly within the healthcare community. Her projects' success attracted the interest of hospitals and other institutions seeking to replicate her strategy. Aisha graciously shared her experiences, providing guidance and resources to individuals embarking on the journey towards greater diversity and inclusion.

Her work started to influence policy at a higher level. Healthcare administrators and legislators frequently turn to her for guidance on enhancing diversity within healthcare systems. Aisha actively participated in panels and committees focused on formulating policies that foster diversity, recognising the need for comprehensive changes to achieve lasting effects.

Aisha's efforts at Mercy Mwongozo led to establishing a diversity and inclusion committee, which provided a platform for ongoing discussions on representation and cultural competence. She was crucial in driving this project and ensuring the hospital's culture and policies aligned with its dedication to diversity.

Aisha's dedication to promoting diversity influenced her work in client advocacy. She ensured that individuals from diverse backgrounds had a voice and that their concerns and needs were recognised and addressed. The focus on client advocacy significantly improved client care and solidified the hospital's connections with the community it served.

The impact of the changes at Mercy Mwongozo extended beyond the staff composition or policy manuals, permeating the hospital's day-to-day interactions. The corridors, waiting areas, and client wards exuded an intellectual curiosity and reverence. Workers demonstrated a heightened understanding and appreciation for diverse cultures, leading to a more cooperative and cohesive professional atmosphere.

Aisha's focus on diversity also had a significant educational influence. Visiting nurses and medical professionals were surrounded by an atmosphere that valued different perspectives and taught them how to provide care with a deep understanding of other cultures. This experience played a vital role in shaping their perspective on healthcare as they advanced in their careers.

Aisha's influence extended beyond the confines of Mercy Mwongozo. Aisha's nursing and healthcare achievements were widely celebrated, but what truly brought her joy was witnessing the tangible impact of her efforts - the smiles on clients' faces, the gratitude from families, and the satisfaction of her colleagues.

Aisha experienced a deep sense of satisfaction as she walked through the hospital, engaging with a team as varied as the clients they cared for. She had transformed her mission into a far-reaching movement that had revolutionised healthcare at Mercy Mwongozo and beyond. Her story showcased the power of an individual to bring about significant transformation and the lasting impact of embracing diversity in every aspect.

Aisha's perspective on diversity will continue to inspire for years. This incident highlighted the importance of recognising that diversity in the healthcare industry goes beyond mere representation. It emphasises the need to enhance the quality of treatment, broaden perspectives, and guarantee compassionate and respectful care for every client. Her impact was a more inclusive, empathetic, and efficient hospital environment, positively affecting future generations of clients and healthcare staff.

Aisha's story ignited inspiration among individuals at Mercy Mwongozo and resonated deeply within the healthcare industry. Her approach to diversity and inclusion is widely recognised as a benchmark for creating more empathetic and thriving healthcare facilities. She was often invited to share her story at various events, sparking intense discussions and deep reflection among healthcare professionals.

The personal stories shared by Aisha's colleagues and clients truly showcased the profound influence of her work. People from various backgrounds expressed how her activism helped them feel respected and empowered. They conveyed their happiness and assurance by recognising and appreciating their unique perspectives. Clients also appreciated the culturally sensitive care they received, leading to better comprehension and compliance with treatment programs.

Aisha's ideas also encompassed community engagement. She understood the importance of embracing diversity and recognised that the hospital should proactively engage with the communities it served to build strong connections. She coordinated health fairs, community dialogues, and outreach programs as platforms for exchanging knowledge and fostering collaboration. These projects helped to make healthcare more accessible and relevant to many people in the community, demystifying it in the process.

Her diligent work significantly enhanced the hospital's hiring and training policies. Aisha worked with the human resources department to develop diversity training programs that included all staff members, not just those directly involved in client care. These programs were designed to increase awareness, question biases, and encourage an inclusive mindset. The employment process was also adjusted to foster a broader candidate pool, showcasing the organisation's dedication to diversity and inclusion at all levels.

Aisha strongly emphasised mentorship and leadership development as she pursued her goal of fostering diversity. She provided guidance and encouragement to several nurses as they pursued their careers in healthcare. Her guidance was instrumental in shaping a new generation of leaders committed to promoting diversity and inclusivity in their professional endeavours.

As Aisha's story spread, other hospitals and healthcare organisations eagerly sought her expertise in implementing similar reforms at their facilities. She embraced a role as a consultant, generously imparting her wealth of knowledge and personal experiences to support and empower others in their endeavours to foster inclusive healthcare environments.

Aisha's impact also extended to the educational sector, sparking significant changes. Following Mercy Mwongozo's example, nursing schools and healthcare training programs started prioritising cultural competence and diversity in their curricula. Aisha often collaborated with these organisations, utilising her practical expertise to enhance the theoretical foundation of healthcare education.

Aisha's dedication to promoting diversity and inclusion influenced healthcare research. Further investigation has been carried out regarding the influence of cultural competence and diversity on healthcare outcomes. The research findings provided other evidence of the importance of Aisha's work, highlighting the need for diversity and inclusion in healthcare environments.

Despite her achievements and recognition, Aisha maintained a modest and determined approach towards her goal. She remained dedicated to promoting diversity and inclusion, constantly striving to enhance and broaden her initiatives. She was a constant presence at local gatherings, in the corridors of Mercy Mwongozo, and wherever her expertise and dedication were needed.

Aisha felt a deep sense of fulfilment as she reflected on her adventure. Her contribution ignited a meaningful conversation, leading to tangible progress and beneficial transformation. She had observed the change in her colleagues' expressions, client feedback, and the evolving culture at Mercy Mwongozo Hospital. However, it is essential to note that she had ignited a movement that has surpassed her contributions, making a lasting impact on healthcare.

Aisha's story served as a powerful reminder of the impact that every person can have in creating a more inclusive and equal society. Her experience showed that enthusiasm, persistence, and bravery make significant change achievable. Her impact would continue to inspire and guide in the coming years, serving as a guiding light for those committed to creating a more diverse, inclusive, and compassionate healthcare sector.

Aisha's contributions to diversity made a significant difference not just in nursing but also in various areas of healthcare. Her approach demonstrated that when healthcare providers from diverse backgrounds work together, they bring expertise and perspectives that enhance the quality of care. This realisation led to a more cohesive approach to client care at Mercy Mwongozo, with teams of doctors, nurses, and allied health workers collaborating more effectively, appreciating each other's diverse perspectives.

Aisha's modifications also led to healthcare practices prioritising the community's needs. The hospital initiated collaborations with local organisations and community leaders to enhance the customisation and adaptability of healthcare initiatives to cater to the needs of the diverse population they served. These collaborations also facilitated a mutual exchange of knowledge, enabling healthcare personnel to better understand the cultural dynamics of the communities they served.

Aisha's commitment to diversity and inclusion had a noticeable impact on the hospital's executive structure. The administration acknowledged the importance of incorporating diverse perspectives into decision-making processes. Consequently, there has been an increase in the number of healthcare professionals from various backgrounds who have taken leadership positions and committees. This adjustment ensured that policies and strategies were crafted with a comprehensive understanding of the distinct requirements of both staff and clients.

Aisha's story has ignited a new surge of research and scholarly exploration into the intersection of healthcare, diversity, and client outcomes. Experts and scholars delved into the long-term effects of her activities, and the findings validated the importance of her endeavours. The study revealed that emphasising diversity and cultural competence significantly enhanced client satisfaction, treatment compliance, and overall healthcare outcomes.

Isha continued to be a role model and a source of inspiration for countless individuals. Her humility, genuineness, and unwavering dedication to her cause garnered the admiration and gratitude of her colleagues, students, and the community. She remained committed to offering advice and guidance, eager to share her wealth of knowledge and personal experiences with individuals striving to make a positive impact.

Aisha's work gained increasing importance as time went on. Mercy Mwongozo Hospital gained recognition for its dedication to inclusivity and as a premier centre for client care. Other institutions thoroughly examined and emulated the hospital's concept, broadening Aisha's visionary idea far beyond its original scope.

Aisha's dedication to diversity and inclusion at Mercy Mwongozo went beyond being a mere tale of organisational transformation. It was a narrative that explored the importance of pushing boundaries, questioning the status quo, and creating an environment where individuals from all walks of life could thrive and make meaningful contributions to the shared goal of delivering exceptional healthcare.

Her experience was a powerful reminder that recognising and valuing diversity in healthcare is crucial for ethical and practical reasons. Aisha's contributions at Mercy Mwongozo and in the broader healthcare community were highly influential, illuminating the path towards a more inclusive, empathetic, and prosperous healthcare system.

Aisha's narrative encompassed far more than the transformations she implemented at Mercy Mwongozo. The focus was on the impact of those changes on clients, healthcare providers, and the community as a whole. Her contributions reached far beyond the confines of the hospital, influencing healthcare practices and policies and leaving a lasting mark on the sector. Aisha's story was a powerful reminder of how an individual's dedication and forward-thinking can profoundly impact the world, gradually transforming it for the better.

CHAPTER 6

Miriam's Moral Predicament

Miriam, an experienced nurse at Mercy Mwongozo, faced a challenging ethical dilemma that would push the boundaries of his values and principles as a healthcare professional. The hospital had implemented a groundbreaking life-extension procedure, a remarkable advancement that could significantly increase lifespan. Nevertheless, this achievement presented Miriam with many ethical dilemmas to navigate.

Miriam found himself deeply conflicted about the impact of the treatment on his overall well-being. Additional time was provided, but at what expense? He observed the provision of this alternative to terminally ill individuals and their families. It was seen by some as a precious chance to prolong their time, to express their unspoken thoughts, and to relish a few extra moments. Some individuals questioned the value of extending life when it meant enduring prolonged suffering.

Miriam's role as a nurse exposed him to these intimate and challenging situations. He engaged in conversations filled with optimism, unease, and ambiguity. His extensive training equipped him with the skills to provide healing and support to those in need. However, he pondered the challenge of guiding clients and their families through a decision that would profoundly impact their lives.

The treatment's ethical implications extended beyond the individuals to the broader healthcare system. Miriam thoroughly analysed resource allocation, financial consequences, and the impact on healthcare service quality. He pondered the delicate balance between prolonging life and preserving its essence.

For Miriam, these moral complexities were not just theoretical concepts but a part of his everyday life. He remembered moments when the therapy enabled families to have additional quality time with their dear ones, leading to beautiful, albeit bittersweet, lasting memories. Nevertheless, there were instances when he pondered if the client's life had been prolonged with the client's utmost welfare in mind.

Miriam's moral dilemmas prompted him to seek guidance from colleagues, ethicists, and mentors. He enthusiastically participated in extensive, sometimes heated discussions regarding the intricacies of medical ethics about treatments that prolong life. These discussions were enlightening, shedding light on the intricacies of the issue and the absence of straightforward resolutions.

Miriam sought answers by engaging directly with clients and families, attentively listening to their stories, concerns, and aspirations. He understood that each case was distinctive, and every decision carried a deeply personal weight. He understood that his role was not to offer solutions but assistance, knowledge, and compassion, no matter the clients' and their families choices.

Miriam's journey through this complex ethical puzzle led to substantial growth in both his personal and professional life. He developed a deeper understanding of the value of life, the importance of respecting clients' choices, and the necessity of providing empathetic and client-focused care. He created the ability to blend his expertise with compassion, recognising that attentive listening and being fully present often yielded the most effective support.

The moral dilemma of Mercy Mwongozo's life-extension treatment reflected contemporary healthcare's broader ethical complexities. Miriam's account highlighted the significance of ongoing discussion, learning, and reforming policies in this area. The importance of preparing healthcare professionals to navigate complex ethical dilemmas was underscored, highlighting the need for them to possess clinical expertise and moral and ethical frameworks to guide their decision-making.

Miriam carried the knowledge he acquired from this incident with him as he continued his work at Mercy Mwongozo. He encouraged deep discussions on ethical matters in nursing school, urging future nurses to confront these complex issues. His story at Mercy Mwongozo was just one of many that reflected the evolving healthcare landscape, where medical breakthroughs often come hand-in-hand with complex ethical dilemmas.

Miriam's journey through his moral dilemma was a testament to the evolving role of nurses in healthcare. It was a poignant reminder that nursing encompasses far more than providing care. It involves navigating the intricate dynamics of life, death, and the ethical complexities of modern medicine. His story became a beacon for others in the industry, showcasing the path of compassion and morality and putting clients at the forefront amidst the ever-growing advancements in medical technology.

Miriam's experiences with the ethical aspects of the new life-extension technique influenced his interactions with colleagues and clients. His thoughtful approach and eagerness to explore moral complexities garnered him acclaim within the institution. Nurses and doctors often sought his advice when faced with complex cases, as they recognised his ability to provide a balanced viewpoint and his deep understanding of the moral aspects of medical care.

The hospital leadership recognised Miriam's exceptional ideas and abilities to navigate these ethical dilemmas. He was invited to join an ethics committee responsible for developing guidelines and procedures for utilising life-extending therapies. Miriam recognised this opportunity to make a significant difference in client care by prioritising ethical considerations in medical decision-making.

During committee discussions, Miriam advocated for policies emphasising client autonomy and quality of life. He highlighted the importance of informed consent, ensuring that clients and their families understand the treatment's consequences before making a choice. His contributions helped create a framework that balanced medical advancements with ethical principles.

Miriam also developed a keen interest in client education. He arranged seminars and information sessions for clients and their families to explore the pros and cons of life-extension therapy. These meetings transformed into forums for open discussion, allowing individuals to freely share their concerns and seek guidance in a supportive environment. Many individuals grappling with challenging choices found solace and insight from Miriam's empathetic method.

Miriam's involvement in the ethics committee and client education reinforced his conviction about effective communication in healthcare. He observed the power of genuine and transparent conversations in alleviating worries, resolving uncertainties, and guiding toward better-informed and morally sound choices. This realisation prompted Miriam to advocate for enhanced communication training in nursing programs, highlighting the importance of effective communication in client care.

Miriam's deep contemplation led him to ponder profound philosophical inquiries regarding the nature of existence, mortality, and the fundamental meaning of healthcare. He was well-versed in various topics, regularly participated in educational events, and engaged in insightful discussions with experts. These findings expanded his understanding and gave him a broader outlook, which he applied to his work at the hospital.

Miriam's contemplation of his ethical dilemma profoundly impacted those in his vicinity. His colleagues were inspired by his commitment to ethical practice, and many started emulating him. The hospital's culture began to embody a heightened sensitivity towards ethical considerations, impacting clinical choices and the overall approach to client care.

Miriam often pondered the significance of his work through his observations. He started with a challenging situation that put his ideas and values to the test. Still, as he progressed, he changed policies, educated clients and families, and fostered an ethical culture. His story showcased the impact of an individual in the intricate realm of healthcare.

Miriam's story at Mercy Mwongozo went beyond simply confronting a moral dilemma; it aimed to inspire others and enhance client care through thoughtful and honest choices. His experience was a powerful reminder of healthcare practitioners' crucial role in navigating modern medicine's ethical landscape. Miriam exemplified a solid commitment to moral principles in navigating the complex landscape of advancing technologies and treatments, providing invaluable support to clients, families, and colleagues.

Miriam's impact in shaping Mercy Mwongozo's ethical framework extended beyond the hospital's confines. Appreciating his wide-reaching ethical dilemmas, he started engaging in more extensive discussions on medical ethics within healthcare forums and online platforms. He shared his insights and personal encounters, contributing to a broader conversation about the impact of life-extension technologies in healthcare.

Miriam's involvement in these forums also connected him with other healthcare professionals facing similar challenges. These connections provide a valuable opportunity for individuals to support and learn from each other. Miriam realised that the ethical challenges in modern medicine were remarkably similar in various healthcare settings, and the importance of a caring and client-focused approach was universally recognised.

At Mercy Mwongozo, Miriam's principles and protocols are seamlessly integrated into the hospital's operations. They served as a valuable guide for ethical decision-making in a range of medical interventions, not just limited to life-extension treatments. The hospital staff appreciated the presence of well-defined guidelines that effectively balanced medical choices with ethical considerations, simplifying the process of making complex decisions.

Miriam also took on the role of a mentor, guiding and supporting young nurses and medical personnel as they navigated the intricate ethical dilemmas of healthcare. He organised regular discussions and case study sessions to explore and debate ethical dilemmas. These seminars have become crucial to Mercy Mwongozo's training and professional development programs, fostering a culture of ethical awareness among the staff.

In addition, Miriam's journey helped him recognise the importance of considering the perspectives of clients and their families when making medical decisions. He advocated for increased client and family participation in discussions about treatment options, ensuring that their perspectives and values were respected. This approach prioritises clients and their families, improves the quality of care, and fosters a more vital trust and understanding between healthcare providers and the individuals they serve.

Miriam's contributions significantly influenced the end-of-life care methods implemented at Mercy Mwongozo. End-of-life decisions were handled with a focus on dignity, client preferences, and quality of life at the hospital. Miriam's contributions helped foster an atmosphere where end-of-life care prioritised quality of life and maintaining dignity throughout the dying process.

Miriam's interest in ethical issues in healthcare led him to collaborate with experts in bioethics and law. They developed comprehensive frameworks to help healthcare providers navigate the moral challenges of modern medicine. These collaborations were phenomenally successful, as other healthcare facilities eagerly adopted the materials and guidelines.

Miriam's profound moral dilemmas drove him to passionately champion the need for enhancements in national policies. He started working with healthcare organisations and policymakers, advocating for policies recognising the ethical considerations of emerging medical technologies and treatments. His research played a significant role in enhancing the recognition of moral considerations in healthcare policy and practice.

Miriam realised that his journey through medical ethics had profoundly impacted his personal life. He had developed a deeper understanding of the human experience, a heightened sensitivity to the delicate nature of life, and a reinvigorated dedication to his role as a career. His experiences reinforced his conviction in the significance of empathy, compassion, and ethical integrity in medical practice.

As Miriam pondered his journey, he realised that his initial dilemma had transformed into a lifelong dedication. He emerged as a strong advocate for ethical healthcare practice, exerting his influence within his immediate community and the broader healthcare landscape.

His story exemplified the power of one individual's dedication to moral principles, igniting transformation and improving the lives of countless individuals.

Miriam's story at Mercy Mwongozo went beyond simply addressing an ethical dilemma; it delved into leadership, advocacy, and the profound impact of ethical mindfulness in healthcare. The text highlighted healthcare practitioners' vital role in navigating modern medicine's complex ethical challenges. Miriam's journey inspired and provided guidance, illuminating a path of moral integrity and compassionate care amidst new challenges and advancements.

Miriam's unwavering commitment to upholding ethical healthcare practices profoundly influenced the broader community surrounding Mercy Mwongozo. He was asked to address students at nearby universities and medical schools about his experiences and insights into the ethical challenges of contemporary healthcare. His speeches ignited a fresh wave of inspiration among a new generation of healthcare workers, instilling a deep appreciation for the importance of ethical considerations in their future careers.

Miriam's work also significantly influenced client advocacy groups. These organisations acknowledged his expertise and perspective and extended invitations for him to engage in discussions and forums. He dedicated himself to championing clients, ensuring their rights and needs were considered in medical decision-making.

Miriam's impact resulted in the establishment of regular ethics forums at Mercy Mwongozo, where employees from various departments convened to engage in thoughtful discussions and deliberations regarding ethical issues in the healthcare field. These forums fostered an atmosphere of open dialogue and cooperative troubleshooting, enabling ethical dilemmas to be addressed from diverse viewpoints.

Miriam actively contributed to developing client education materials that included sections on ethical considerations in medical care. These resources helped clients and their families navigate the complex world of healthcare decisions, providing them with knowledge and support.

He extended his advocacy for ethical healthcare to global platforms as well. Miriam collaborated with international health organisations to develop moral principles that can be applied in diverse healthcare environments worldwide. His work profoundly impacted a global scale, reshaping the perspectives of healthcare practitioners worldwide regarding ethical dilemmas.

As Miriam continued his endeavours, he often reflected on his journey to this moment. He started with a significant personal issue and turned it into an opportunity to impact the healthcare industry positively. His story showcased an individual's immense impact on shaping policies and procedures that positively affect clients and healthcare professionals.

Miriam's unwavering dedication to upholding ethical standards in healthcare procedures was duly noted. He received recognition and awards for his contributions. However, Miriam found true joy in witnessing the tangible effects of his work - the grateful smiles of clients, the considerate actions of his colleagues, and the transformative policies of healthcare organisations.

His journey highlighted the importance of ongoing learning and adaptability in healthcare. The industry was constantly evolving, presenting fresh challenges and ethical dilemmas. Miriam embraced the ever-changing nature of his work, always dedicated to staying knowledgeable and attuned to the dynamic healthcare industry. Miriam had transcended his role as a nurse in the Mercy Mwongozo halls. He had become a guiding figure, inspiring others with his wisdom and setting a high standard of ethical conduct. His story inspired his colleagues to be as diligent and dedicated to moral behaviour as he was.

Miriam's experience at Mercy Mwongozo showcased the profound intersection of healthcare and ethics. The text highlighted the crucial importance of healthcare practitioners in navigating the complex ethical challenges of modern medicine. His continuous learning and personal growth journey have been a source of inspiration and guidance, illuminating the path of moral integrity and compassionate care in the dynamic healthcare field.

CHAPTER 7

Zara Takes the Lead

Zara's journey at Mercy Mwongozo Hospital transformed remarkably, evolving from a dedicated bedside nurse to a forward-thinking healthcare executive. Her journey was marked by an unwavering commitment to providing excellent client care and a growing awareness of the potential impact she could have beyond the confines of the hospital.

Zara was known for her exceptional ability to connect with clients during the early stages of her career. Her compassion and expertise garnered her clients' and colleagues' respect. However, as she delved into the intricacies of healthcare, Zara became aware of the broader issues impacting client care. She noticed recurring challenges, inefficiencies, and gaps in healthcare delivery that often hindered the providing the best possible care.

Zara started to assume additional responsibilities outside of her nursing duties, driven by her aspiration to have a broader impact. She actively participated in hospital committees, contributing valuable insights and suggestions to enhance client care services. Her extensive nursing experience provided her with a unique perspective firmly rooted in the practicalities of client care.

She was tasked with completely revamping the client flow mechanism in the emergency department. Zara's methodical and client-centric approach prioritised reducing wait times and enhancing the client experience. The success of this project not only improved client care but highlighted Zara's exceptional leadership skills and ability to solve problems effectively.

Appreciating Zara's potential, the hospital administration encouraged her to further her education in healthcare administration. Zara's education expanded her perspectives, equipping her with the knowledge and skills to make a meaningful difference. She delved into the intricacies of healthcare policy, finance, and administration, gaining a comprehensive grasp of the healthcare system.

Zara's understanding of healthcare grew in tandem with her career. She passionately advocated for client-centred care models, placing clients' needs and experiences at the forefront of healthcare delivery. She spearheaded initiatives to integrate client feedback into the evolution of hospital services, guaranteeing that the client's perspective was consistently acknowledged and valued.

Zara's leadership focused on cultivating a constant improvement and innovation culture rather than simply executing changes. She motivated and inspired her nursing colleagues, urging them to be proactive and think creatively when addressing healthcare challenges. Mercy Mwongozo's nursing workforce flourished under her guidance, becoming more engaged and bolder and making significant contributions to the quality of treatment.

Her impact expanded beyond the hospital as she presented at regional and national healthcare conferences. In these forums, Zara passionately championed policies and practices that supported the nursing profession and improved client care. Her speeches and presentations were captivating, drawing from her vast nursing experience and perspectives as a healthcare leader.

Zara's journey reached its pinnacle when she was promoted to a prestigious leadership role at Mercy Mwongozo. In this role, she shaped policy, influenced organisational culture, and made substantial progress in healthcare service. She had a thoughtful leadership style, consistently acknowledging her team's contributions and fostering collaboration.

Zara's story showcased the capacity of nurses to take charge and transform the healthcare industry. Her journey from bedside nursing to healthcare leadership was shaped by courage, perseverance, and dedication to clients' well-being. She challenged societal norms and paved the way for future nursing leaders.

Zara's new work was guided by the principles that had shaped her as a nurse: a deep understanding of others, a genuine concern for their well-being, and an unwavering focus on providing the best possible care for her clients. Her journey served as a potent reminder that nurses' insights and experiences play a vital role in shaping the future of healthcare. Mercy Mwongozo was fortunate to have Zara, a forward-thinking individual who consistently motivated and drove progress in healthcare.

Zara's visionary leadership brought a fresh perspective to Mercy Mwongozo's management. Her extensive practical experience as a nurse gave her a profound understanding of the challenges clients and healthcare providers face. This understanding became the foundation of her leadership philosophy, which focused on compassion, effectiveness, and creativity in healthcare provision.

Zara's primary focus in her new role was to enhance communication between different departments within the hospital. She understood that providing excellent client care necessitated smooth coordination among other departments. Thanks to her guidance, the hospital implemented innovative communication protocols and collaborative technologies, resulting in enhanced coordination and decreased client care delays.

She was focused on enhancing staff development and promoting well-being. Zara had a deep understanding of the challenges that come with burnout and stress among healthcare personnel. She supported initiatives that promoted the mental and emotional well-being of the staff. The programs available encompass a variety of wellness courses, stress management sessions, and initiatives aimed at fostering a healthy work-life balance.

Zara played a crucial role in expanding Mercy Mwongozo's community outreach efforts. She believed the hospital was responsible for serving the entire community, extending beyond its physical boundaries. The hospital implemented various community health initiatives under her guidance, such as free screening programs, health education seminars, and collaborations with local schools to promote health and wellness.

Zara was a strong proponent of nurse leadership in healthcare policy in her broader advocacy efforts. She proposed that nurses were uniquely positioned to make valuable contributions to healthcare policymaking because of their firsthand experience and client-focused mindset. Her activism brought attention to the critical role of nurses in shaping healthcare policies at both the state and national levels.

Zara faced numerous challenges on her journey to becoming a leader. She often found herself dealing with intricate bureaucracies and facing resistance to change. Nevertheless, her unwavering commitment and focus on her mission allowed her to overcome these obstacles. She inspired many in the healthcare industry, showcasing how nurses could ascend to positions in the city and make a significant impact.

Under Zara's guidance, Mercy Mwongozo Hospital experienced significant improvements in client satisfaction and staff morale. Her innovative methods and cutting-edge programs revolutionised care quality while optimising hospital operations. Zara believes that true success lies in the stories of clients whose lives were improved by the treatment and the personnel who rediscovered their purpose and passion in their work.

As Zara reflected on her journey, she came to understand that her progression from bedside nursing to healthcare leadership was not just a personal achievement but also a reflection of the evolving role of nursing in healthcare. She had shown that nurses' extensive understanding of client care and healthcare systems were valuable assets in leadership roles.

Zara's experience at Mercy Mwongozo was a thought-provoking journey that challenged societal norms and reshaped traditional expectations. The focus was on the potential for an individual to transform a healthcare institution and shape the broader healthcare landscape. Her journey continues to captivate and invigorate, highlighting the capacity of nursing professionals to take charge and bring fresh ideas to the dynamic healthcare industry. Zara's journey to healthcare leadership was a remarkable tale of personal triumph, inspiring aspiring nurse leaders. Her experience showcased the extraordinary capacity of nurses to go beyond their traditional responsibilities and make significant contributions to the highest levels of hospital administration.

Zara's influential position allowed her to have a direct impact on policies that shape client care. She dedicated herself to ensuring the success of these policies while prioritising the needs and values of clients and staff. She consistently sought input from various individuals before reaching conclusions, fostering a collaborative atmosphere.

Zara's notable achievement was establishing a client advisory group at Mercy Mwongozo. This council, comprised of individuals previously receiving treatment and their loved ones, offered invaluable perspectives on the hospital's client experience. Their contribution was crucial in developing client care policy, ensuring the hospital's services aligned with clients' real needs.

Zara was also intrigued by leveraging technology to enhance healthcare delivery. She managed the implementation of advanced data analytics in hospital operations, which helped identify trends in client care, predict resource needs, and improve the facility's overall effectiveness. Mercy Mwongozo established itself as a cutting-edge institution in the healthcare industry due to its visionary approach to incorporating technology.

Her dedication to public health projects expanded her impact on the broader community. Zara understood the interconnectedness of personal well-being and the well-being of the community. She partnered with public health organisations to tackle chronic disease management, mental health, and health education issues. These programs not only enhance health outcomes but also play a role in fostering more robust and thriving communities.

Zara remained grounded in her nursing background, even as she took on a leadership role. She persistently championed nurses, ensuring their perspectives were acknowledged in domains traditionally dominated by other healthcare professionals. She passionately supported nursing education, advocating for curricula aligned with the changing healthcare landscape.

Zara's leadership style was characterised by understanding, assertiveness, and foresight. She was highly regarded for her exceptional listening skills, ability to understand others, and unwavering determination when faced with challenging decisions.

Her leadership demonstrated a thoughtful approach that prioritised clients' needs while considering the long-term implications for healthcare.

Zara's contributions influenced the culture at Mercy Mwongozo. The hospital gained a reputation for its progressive and inclusive approach to healthcare. Employees at all levels experienced a heightened sense of engagement and appreciation, improving the quality of client care. Zara had cultivated a culture that embraced and celebrated creativity and brilliance.

Zara excelled in healthcare, gaining recognition as a highly sought-after speaker and consultant. She utilised these forums to generously share her vast knowledge and valuable experiences, advocating passionately for healthcare reform. Her speeches and courses have been a source of inspiration and guidance for many healthcare professionals.

Zara stayed down-to-earth and maintained strong connections with her colleagues despite her busy schedule. She regularly explored the corridors of Mercy Mwongozo, engaging with the staff and clients and staying informed about the everyday experiences on the hospital floor. These connections exposed her to the daily challenges and successes of client care, fueling her passion for creating an impact.

Zara's experience showcased the evolving nature of healthcare leadership. She embodied a fresh leader who went beyond mere administrator and genuinely cared about others. Her story was a powerful testament to the idea that diverse professional experiences, including nursing, enhance the effectiveness of healthcare leadership.

Zara's impact expanded in the subsequent years. Her concepts at Mercy Mwongozo served as models for other hospitals. Her story was a powerful inspiration, motivating a new wave of nurses to pursue positions of influence and proving that nurses possess the drive and ambition to reach the pinnacle of healthcare leadership.

Zara's time at Mercy Mwongozo went beyond mere professional growth; it was a remarkable display of visionary leadership that significantly changed the healthcare industry. The nursing profession has the incredible power to shape and determine the future of healthcare. Zara was a remarkable individual, serving as both a leader and a visionary who completely transformed the healthcare industry. Her journey from nursing to healthcare leadership has left an indelible mark on the field.

Zara's impact and leadership at Mercy Mwongozo started to align with more extensive efforts to enhance healthcare services nationwide. She enthusiastically participated in national healthcare reform, offering her expertise and perspectives to discussions that shaped future healthcare legislation. Her expertise in articulating the needs and concerns of frontline healthcare workers was indispensable in these reform initiatives.

Mercy Mwongozo Hospital emerged as a trailblazer in client-centred care during Zara's tenure, introducing groundbreaking procedures that other hospitals and healthcare institutions subsequently adopted. She was pivotal in initiatives focusing on medical care and promoting overall health and wellness. These initiatives showcased Zara's belief that healthcare should be approached proactively rather than reactively. Her commitment to delivering exceptional healthcare was evident in her efforts to foster research and development at Mercy Mwongozo. Zara fostered collaborations with research institutions and pharmaceutical businesses to introduce state-of-the-art therapies and technologies to the hospital. These partnerships improved client outcomes and established Mercy Mwongozo as a leader in medical innovation.

Zara was deeply dedicated to the growth and advancement of her employees. She prioritised the importance of continuous learning and skill development within the hospital's culture. Her contributions in this field improved the standard of client care and boosted staff morale and career growth.

In addition, Zara's leadership style was known for its welcoming and accessible approach. She valued being accessible to her team and consistently demonstrated a willingness to hear their concerns and ideas. This approach fostered a sense of trust and mutual respect, leading to a united and motivated team.

Her leadership career served as a great inspiration to many young professionals, especially women in the healthcare field. Zara emerged as an exemplary figure, showcasing that they could be achieved through diligent work, dedication, and a pursuit of excellence. She actively engaged in mentorship programs, providing guidance and support to individuals aspiring to leadership positions in healthcare.

Zara's journey transcended the conventional tale of career progression. It revolved around tapping into the power of nursing to impact healthcare as a whole significantly. Highlighting nurses' unique insights, she demonstrated the valuable perspectives they offer to healthcare administrators. Her journey also emphasised the importance of having a variety of perspectives in positions of power. Zara's nursing expertise brought a distinct range of experiences and perspectives to the decision-making table, leading to the development of more comprehensive and client-focused healthcare policies and practices.

Zara's unwavering dedication and commitment have profoundly impacted Mercy Mwongozo, leaving a lasting legacy. The hospital's performance under her direction became a prime example of effective healthcare administration, showcasing nurses' significant influence in leadership positions.

Zara's story highlighted the evolving role of nurses in healthcare. The text emphasised the significance of the healthcare system, acknowledging and harnessing the immense potential of nurses in leadership positions. Her remarkable transition from bedside nursing to healthcare leadership is a guiding light for the nursing profession, offering a clear path for aspiring nurse leaders who desire to bring about meaningful change in healthcare.

CHAPTER 8

John's Quiet Struggle

John, a caring nurse at Mercy Mwongozo, was widely recognised for his unwavering commitment to his clients. However, behind his composed exterior, he was engaged in a silent struggle - a struggle with his emotional well-being that mirrored the challenges faced by numerous individuals under his care. John's journey through this personal challenge enhanced his comprehension of mental health within the realm of healthcare.

Every day, as he encountered individuals grappling with diverse mental illnesses, John couldn't help but see a mirror of his struggles in theirs. He attentively absorbed their stories, understanding their pain and confusion in a way that only someone who had experienced similar emotions could. He was an exceptional carer due to his profound empathy, although it sometimes made distinguishing between his professional obligations and personal emotions difficult.

Over time, John began to recognise his struggles with mental health. The constant exposure to pain, the demanding atmosphere of the hospital, and the emotional burden of tending to others started to take a heavy toll on him. At first, he disregarded his emotions as mere hazards of his profession. However, over time, he realised that what he was experiencing was more than just ordinary stress. It was a challenging struggle that demanded attention.

Despite his understanding of mental health challenges, John struggled to ask for help. Mental health was often stigmatised, especially among healthcare workers, who were expected to be strong and resilient. John found it challenging to overcome the perception that acknowledging his mental health concerns was a professional vulnerability.

However, John had a moment of realisation when he understood that his personal experiences could be a source of strength instead of a weakness. His battle with mental illness gave him a distinct viewpoint on client care, especially when it comes to tending to his client's emotional and psychological well-being. This realisation inspired John to seek help bravely.

Professional therapy, self-care, and the support of colleagues and friends were instrumental in John's journey towards healing. As he navigated his struggles, he started speaking out about the importance of mental health care for healthcare practitioners. He initiated initiatives within the hospital to enhance mental health awareness, urging his colleagues to prioritise their well-being.

His efforts established a hospital staff support system, offering access to counselling services, mental health days, and wellness programs. John's contributions in this field have played a significant role in fostering a more inclusive and supportive work environment, consequently diminishing the negative perception surrounding mental health within the healthcare sector.

John's unique perspective influenced his approach to client care. He developed a heightened awareness of his client's mental health concerns, championing a holistic approach to healthcare that encompassed both physical and psychological well-being. He began to adopt a more comprehensive approach to client treatment, considering the emotional and psychological factors contributing to recovery.

John also became involved in community outreach programs promoting mental health awareness. He openly shared his story, eventually becoming a champion for mental health. His openness and willingness to share his struggles helped dismantle barriers and inspire others to seek help.

John's battle with mental illness and his journey toward recovery had a profound impact on how mental health was perceived and addressed at Mercy Mwongozo. His struggles sparked a wave of positive change, not only within the hospital but also in the broader community.

His story was a powerful reminder of the hidden challenges that healthcare professionals face. The significance of support services and open discussions on mental health in the healthcare sector was underscored. John's journey showcased the importance of embracing vulnerability and recognising the equal importance of mental and physical health.

John's struggle with mental illness transcended the boundaries of his own experience, becoming a powerful narrative of growth and optimism. It sheds light on a frequently neglected aspect of carer well-being, underscoring the importance of mental health for those who dedicate their lives to caring for others. John's story became an integral part of the stories at Mercy Mwongozo, contributing to a more compassionate, empathetic, and comprehensive approach to healthcare.

John's dedication and hard work played a crucial role in shaping the culture of Mercy Mwongozo Hospital. His openness regarding his challenges motivated others to acknowledge and confront their mental health concerns. Discussions surrounding mental health became increasingly common among employees, fostering a warm and empathetic work environment.

Appreciating the importance of John's endeavours, the hospital administration integrated mental health into their comprehensive wellness programs. They implemented regular mental health assessments for employees, offering support and access to resources for those who require it. This forward-thinking approach represented a significant shift from the passive approach previously employed in healthcare settings.

John also coordinated workshops and seminars in partnership with local mental health organisations. These gatherings offered healthcare professionals and the Mwongozo public valuable information and resources. John's contributions were instrumental in changing societal perceptions of mental health, emphasising that seeking treatment is a display of resilience rather than vulnerability.

His impact also reached the realm of client care. John worked closely with the hospital's medical staff to integrate mental health assessments into the standard care protocols. He advocated for a holistic approach to treatment, recognising the importance of clients' cognitive and emotional well-being and overall health. This approach led to more thorough care plans and enhanced client outcomes.

In addition, John's personal experience gave him a distinct viewpoint on the client experience, specifically for individuals dealing with mental health issues. He emerged as a crucial consultant in advancing client-centred care models that integrated mental health as a significant element. His ideas led to a healthcare environment that was both compassionate and effective.

John's efforts had a profound influence on the entire institution. The employees' spirits were lifted as they experienced greater appreciation and assistance. This positive work environment improved client care, as staff members were more equipped to handle the emotional challenges of their roles.

John's powerful story of overcoming challenges and channelling his experience to make a difference deeply resonated with everyone at Mercy Mwongozo. He emerged as a symbol of resilience, a testament to the importance of voicing one's thoughts, and a champion for the well-being of mental health. His journey was a poignant reminder that even healthcare professionals are not immune to personal struggles.

John's dedication to his cause has propelled him to become a prominent figure in mental health within healthcare settings. He frequently reflected on his journey, appreciative of the knowledge he had gained and satisfied with the impact he had helped to create. His narrative was more than just a tale of personal triumph; it also showcased how individual challenges can be turned into chances to impact the world significantly.

John's impact at Mercy Mwongozo and beyond was a captivating narrative emphasising the significance of mental health in healthcare. The text highlighted the importance of healthcare organisations placing a strong emphasis on the well-being of their employees to ensure the delivery of optimal treatment to clients. John's journey from a silent battle to a powerful advocate for change has been a source of inspiration and hope for many in the healthcare field. His story is a guiding light for those seeking to make a difference.

John's influence extended beyond Mercy Mwongozo Hospital and the broader healthcare community. His endeavours and advocacy work gained recognition among healthcare organisations and mental health advocacy groups. He was invited to speak at national conferences and forums, where he shared his story and the critical transformations he had achieved at Mercy Mwongozo.

During these engagements, John discussed the importance of healthcare professionals acknowledging and tackling mental health concerns. He highlighted the significance of taking a holistic approach to mental well-being in healthcare environments, recognising that the well-being of carers directly affects the quality of client care. His comments often resonated with his listeners, a significant number of whom were healthcare professionals grappling with their mental well-being.

At Mercy Mwongozo, the impact of John's actions became apparent. His expertise in developing worker wellness programs became a benchmark for other hospitals. Regular mental health check-ins, access to counselling services, and stress management training became commonplace. Staff at the hospital noticed a significant improvement in their overall well-being, leading to a remarkable boost in client care and staff interactions.

John was crucial in integrating mental health education into Mercy Mwongozo's nurse and doctor training programs. He worked alongside educational leaders to develop curricula incorporating modules on self-care, mental health awareness, and strategies for managing stress and burnout. His dedication ensured that the upcoming generation of healthcare professionals was better equipped to handle the psychological challenges of their profession.

The hospital's approach to client care showcased the profound influence of John's endeavours. There was a strong focus on the cognitive and psychological aspects of healing. Healthcare teams have started incorporating mental health exams into routine client evaluations. John was actively involved in collaborating with these teams, offering his knowledge and support in creating treatment plans that considered clients' holistic needs, encompassing both their physical and mental well-being.

John's lobbying led to partnerships with mental health organisations, paving the way for joint initiatives and community engagement programs. These collaborations helped to increase awareness about mental health issues, decrease stigma, and motivate more individuals to seek treatment.

In addition, John's journey and the improvements he advocated for at Mercy Mwongozo started to influence discussions on higher-level policies. Healthcare policymakers began acknowledging the importance of carer mental health, leading to conversations about implementing similar wellness programs nationwide in hospitals and healthcare institutions.

John experienced a profound sense of meaning in his personal life. He viewed his struggle with mental health as a chance to impact the lives of others rather than a burden. His journey had completed its cycle, transitioning from battling his hidden struggle in isolation to leading a movement that prioritised mental well-being.

John's story ignited inspiration and motivation in those around him. His colleagues at Mercy Mwongozo, motivated by the changes he had implemented, started to play a more proactive role in promoting mental health within their professional and personal circles. John had initiated a movement that was now being continued by others, impacting the healthcare community.

Reflecting on his journey, John experienced a profound sense of achievement. He had transformed his quiet battle into a powerful catalyst for change, impacting not only his existence but also the lives of numerous individuals. His story showcased the strength of being open and the importance of prioritising mental well-being on par with physical well-being.

At Mercy Mwongozo, John's story was a powerful testament to the profound impact of addressing mental health in healthcare. It showcased the potential for transformation, optimism, and the implications of prioritising mental well-being. The text highlighted the importance of empathy towards oneself and others and the significant influence that empathetic care can have on the healthcare system. John's experience had a profound impact, not only on himself but also on the way healthcare professionals approached mental health. His influence has created a lasting legacy of heightened awareness, increased support, and improved understanding.

John's story had a profound impact on driving change beyond the confines of the hospital. The advocacy and activities of His Mercy Mwongozo have captured the attention of many health organisations and educational institutes. They aimed to replicate John's successful mental health support and awareness models.

He began collaborating with universities and nursing schools, highlighting the importance of incorporating mental health education into healthcare curricula. John enthusiastically shared his experiences through guest lectures and workshops, passionately advocating for the inclusion of mental health awareness and self-care skills in healthcare curricula. His involvement profoundly impacted the future of healthcare professionals, equipping them with the necessary resources to address their mental well-being effectively.

The broader medical community started to acknowledge the importance of John's work. Despite receiving numerous awards and recognition, John found great satisfaction in observing a significant shift in attitudes towards mental health within the healthcare profession. The impact of Mercy Mwongozo's changes was now felt by hospitals and healthcare institutions nationwide.

John also delved into research studies exploring the effects of mental health initiatives on the efficiency and standard of client care among healthcare workers. His research provided valuable insights that underscored the importance of mental well-being in the healthcare profession. These findings promoted a more comprehensive approach to healthcare, where the significance of mental health is on par with physical health.

John's contributions left a lasting impression at Mercy Mwongozo. The hospital staff operated with increased unity and effectiveness as they became more aware of and empathetic towards each other's psychological well-being. The hospital set a precedent for other organisations striving to create a more welcoming and conducive work environment for their employees. John's journey with mental health had evolved from a quiet struggle to a passionate and determined call for transformation. He had challenged the prevailing attitudes towards mental health in healthcare, sparking a dialogue far beyond Mercy Mwongozo Hospital's confines.

John maintained a modest and approachable demeanour throughout his professional journey, consistently open to listening and providing support. He became a guiding figure for numerous individuals, generously imparting his wisdom and insights while offering unwavering support during their challenges. His journey served as a source of inspiration, showcasing that even in the most challenging circumstances, there is always room for hope and the potential for personal growth.

John's work profoundly impacted the healthcare system, fostering a culture of compassion, understanding, and achievement. His dedication to promoting mental health transformed the environment at Mercy Mwongozo and sparked a movement within the broader healthcare community. John's story brought to mind the strength of acknowledging one's imperfections and the profound influence an individual can have on effecting widespread transformation. Over the years, John has continued to be a prominent advocate for mental health awareness. His unwavering commitment to the cause was a constant source of inspiration, driving positive change. His story went beyond a personal account; it served as an inspiration and a call to action for healthcare professionals and institutions to recognise the importance of mental health in healthcare.

CHAPTER 9

Grace's Advocacy for the Elderly

Grace, an experienced nurse at Mercy Mwongozo Hospital, has always been fascinated by geriatric care. Throughout her nursing career, she gained firsthand experience of the unique joys and difficulties of caring for older people. This passion developed into a solid commitment to improving and revolutionising geriatric care.

Her commitment to older people was rooted in the belief that they deserved more than medical attention—they deserved to be treated with dignity, empathy, and respect. Grace appreciated the unique backgrounds, experiences, and stories of her elderly clients, seeing them as individuals rather than just a list of physical ailments. This perspective motivated her to surpass the limits of nursing, dedicating herself to enhancing the well-being of her elderly clients.

Grace highlighted a crucial challenge in geriatric care: the need for specialised training among healthcare providers. To tackle this issue, she initiated a series of training sessions at Mercy Mwongozo that specifically targeted the distinct needs of elderly clients. These workshops focused on chronic illness management, the psychological consequences of ageing, and providing compassionate end-of-life care.

Her dedication to making a difference went beyond the hospital's boundaries. Grace dedicated her time to collaborating with local community centres and nursing homes, striving to enhance the standard of care in these environments. She coordinated community outreach programs to educate families and caregivers on providing proper care for their elderly loved ones.

Mercy Mwongozo's comprehensive geriatric care program was a key focus of Grace's efforts. This program utilised diverse expertise to develop personalised care plans for elderly individuals, involving doctors, nurses, dietitians, and therapists. The program achieved remarkable success, improving client outcomes and setting a new benchmark for geriatric care in the hospital.

Grace also advocated for policy reforms. She tirelessly campaigned for increased funding in senior care at both the state and national levels. She dedicated her efforts to raising awareness about the growing needs of the ageing population and the importance of implementing more comprehensive and compassionate care programs.

Her passion for senior care was infectious. Mercy Mwongozo's colleagues were captivated by her enthusiasm and started to view geriatric care from a fresh angle. Many individuals rallied behind her cause, forming a formidable group committed to enhancing the well-being of elderly individuals.

Grace was instrumental in establishing support groups for the family members of elderly clients. These groups offered a platform for individuals to exchange their experiences, provide assistance, and gain knowledge on navigating the complexities of caring for ageing family members. Many families found the support groups invaluable, offering them knowledge, solace, and a sense of belonging.

Grace also highlighted the importance of mental health in geriatric care. She integrated mental health assessments into the senior care program, ensuring that the emotional and psychological needs of elderly clients were addressed. Her comprehensive approach to aged care showcased her understanding that optimal health in old age requires attention to both physical and mental well-being.

Grace's dedication to advocating for older people and her impressive accomplishments gained her recognition beyond the confines of Mercy Mwongozo. She gained recognition in geriatric nursing, and her expertise led to numerous invitations to speak at conferences and seminars. Her perspectives and insights enriched the discourse on aged care, leaving a lasting impact on healthcare professionals nationwide.

Grace's profound influence on geriatric care was evident in the lives of countless older clients and their families as she tirelessly pursued her work. She had transformed her passion into a movement, reshaping the way people view and provide care for older people. She shared a touching narrative of empathy, perseverance, and a drive to bring about positive change in the lives of older people.

Grace's career in old advocacy was a testament to her unwavering dedication to the dignity and well-being of older people. Her work at Mercy Mwongozo and elsewhere showcased the remarkable impact that a single person can have on transforming a specific area of healthcare. Her influence was a kinder, more thorough, and highly regarded approach to geriatric care, which became a blueprint for future healthcare professionals.

Grace's commitment to geriatric care became a leading force in the field. She understood the importance of valuing and respecting the opinions and experiences of older people in providing quality care. She initiated a Mercy Mwongozo program involving older clients in care planning. This approach empowered individuals and gave healthcare providers a deeper understanding of their needs and preferences.

Her work in geriatric care involves conducting research. Grace collaborated with academic institutions to explore the effectiveness of different strategies for aged care. The study sought to understand the most effective techniques in aged care, ranging from managing chronic diseases to supporting mental health. The research findings made a significant contribution to the field of geriatric care and had a widespread impact on care practices beyond Mercy Mwongozo.

Grace understood the importance of technology in enhancing the well-being of older adults as she worked towards improving geriatric care. She strongly supported using technology to monitor and manage the health of elderly individuals. Telehealth services facilitated remote client monitoring, while digital platforms enhanced communication between clients, families, and healthcare practitioners.

Grace's dedication to geriatric care extended to her tireless efforts in championing the rights of older people in healthcare settings. She passionately opposed ageism in healthcare, challenging biases and promoting the belief that elderly individuals deserve equal access to quality care. Her campaign highlighted the frequently neglected problem of age discrimination in healthcare.

Grace's work in geriatric care had a profound influence. Significant progress was made in enhancing the level of care provided to elderly clients at Mercy Mwongozo. Grace's unwavering commitment and enthusiasm motivated the staff to gain a deeper appreciation for the intricacies of elderly care.

In addition, Grace's geriatric care programs started to influence healthcare system policies. Her dedication and research played a crucial role in developing legislation that aimed to improve the well-being of older people. These policies encompassed a boost in funding for senior care programs, enhanced training for healthcare personnel in geriatric care, and a heightened focus on research in this field.

Grace's work advanced, and she became a mentor to numerous nurses and healthcare workers. Her expertise inspired them to focus on elderly care and approach their work with equal empathy and commitment. Grace guided and supported a new wave of healthcare professionals dedicated to providing exceptional care for older people.

Grace's story at Mercy Mwongozo revolved around her capacity to ignite transformation and foster a shared transformation in the perception and provision of senior care. She had left a lasting impact on geriatric care that would endure for years to come.

Her journey was a captivating demonstration of how determination and passion can result in significant advancements in a particular healthcare domain. Grace's story highlighted the importance of championing marginalised populations within the healthcare system. Her work in geriatric care was a shining example of compassion and comprehensive care for older people, providing them with hope and dignity.

Grace's influence on geriatric care expanded as her methods and programs became renowned for their excellence in senior care. She was invited to collaborate with other hospitals and healthcare institutes, offering her expertise and assisting them in advancing geriatric care programs. Her approach, with a focus on dignity and holistic care, was starting to revolutionise the treatment of elderly clients in various healthcare settings.

Her passion for geriatric care drove her to advocate strongly for legislative reforms that would improve the lives of the elderly beyond the confines of hospitals. Grace understood the importance of extending care beyond the confines of one's home. She dedicated herself to tirelessly improving public spaces, transportation, and housing to create a more inclusive and accommodating environment for older people.

Grace understood the importance of receiving support from family and carers in her ongoing efforts to enhance geriatric care. She facilitated workshops and support groups for the families of elderly clients, equipping them with the necessary tools and knowledge to provide improved care for their loved ones. These programs helped families gain a deeper understanding of the ageing process, navigate the challenges of caregiving, and make well-informed decisions regarding the care of their elderly loved ones.

Grace's approach to aged care encompassed end-of-life care. She advocated for a compassionate and respectful approach to end-of-life care, ensuring clients' wishes and dignity were honoured. Her contributions in this field brought comfort and tranquillity to numerous clients and their families, revolutionising how end-of-life care is perceived and provided.

Grace's work in geriatric care profoundly influenced educational programs for healthcare workers. She collaborated with academic institutions to develop comprehensive geriatric care curriculums, acknowledging the importance of specialised training in aged care. These programs emphasised older people's unique medical, psychological, and social needs, equipping healthcare professionals to provide more impactful and empathetic care.

Her actions profoundly impacted the lives of numerous elderly individuals, both at Mercy Mwongozo and in the broader community. The older clients under their care experienced improved client outcomes, including lower rates of hospital readmissions and a higher overall quality of life.

Grace's dedication to geriatric care brought about a significant change in the culture at Mercy Mwongozo. The medical personnel gained a deeper appreciation and comprehension of older people due to her passion and dedication. This cultural shift enhanced the overall atmosphere of the hospital, creating a friendlier and more empathetic environment for elderly clients.

Grace's work advanced, and she became a highly regarded figure in senior care. She is known for her groundbreaking ideas and sincere dedication to the well-being of older people. Her journey from Mercy Mwongozo nurse to major champion for senior care has been a source of inspiration for many.

Her story was a powerful reminder of the importance of specialised care for older people. The text highlighted the significance of healthcare systems being able to adjust and meet the increasing needs of an ageing population. Grace's impact on ageing care was marked by her compassionate approach, innovative ideas, and unwavering commitment to excellence.

Grace's time at Mercy Mwongozo went beyond mere professional achievements; it involved revolutionising the elderly care landscape. Her work was truly inspiring, showcasing the profound impact that compassionate and devoted care can have on the lives of older people. Her journey left a lasting impact on the world of healthcare, inspiring and guiding those dedicated to improving and honouring the lives of older people.

Grace's unwavering commitment to geriatric care profoundly impacted the practice and public perception of senior care. Her unique perspective, highlighting the importance of mental, emotional, and social aspects of ageing and physical well-being, changed the conversation surrounding elderly care. It was now seen as more than managing the effects of ageing but as a chance to enhance the well-being of older individuals.

The inclusion of more segments on geriatric care in medical conferences and seminars, often featuring Grace as a prominent speaker, demonstrated a notable change in perception. Her speeches, brimming with wisdom from her personal experiences, provided practical strategies for improving aged care and underscored the importance of treating elderly individuals with dignity and honour.

The geriatric care program that Grace had advocated for at Mercy Mwongozo became a shining example of client-centred care. The program's success led to its adoption by other hospital departments, transforming the overall client care approach. This all-encompassing approach successfully addressed clients' needs with multiple chronic conditions, a common occurrence in geriatric care.

Grace also recognised the importance of technology in enhancing geriatric care. She focused on integrating technological solutions to improve the quality of life for elderly clients. This encompassed telemedicine services that enhanced healthcare accessibility for elders and computerised monitoring systems that facilitated proactive management of chronic illnesses.

Grace's endeavours also involved establishing a community focused on senior care. She coordinated events that brought together older individuals, their loved ones, and medical professionals. These activities allowed individuals to exchange experiences, assist, and forge new connections. They enhanced older people's sense of community, effectively countering the isolation often accompanying ageing.

Grace's expertise in geriatric care also led to her involvement in policy matters. She advocated for more significant financial support and additional resources for programs dedicated to caring for older people. Her contributions helped to enhance policy measures that expanded healthcare access for older people, especially in underserved communities.

Grace's work advanced, and she emerged as a mentor and role model for numerous individuals in the healthcare field. Her narrative showcased the power of passion and dedication in achieving significant advancements in the field. By sharing her knowledge and passion, she inspired a new generation of healthcare workers to focus on senior care.

Grace's contributions at Mercy Mwongozo and the broader healthcare community have been profoundly impacted. She revolutionised geriatric care, propelling it to the forefront of healthcare debates and procedures. Her dedication to the well-being of older people improved their quality of care and brought attention to their unique needs and challenges.

Grace's narrative transcended mere professional achievement and served as a testament to an individual's profound impact on enhancing a critical aspect of healthcare. Her story is inspiring, showcasing the importance of empathy, creativity, and advocacy in elderly care. Grace's contributions have profoundly impacted the field of geriatric care, establishing a lasting legacy that will shape the care of elderly individuals for generations to come.

CHAPTER 10

The Breaking Point of Noah

Noah, a committed and empathetic Mercy Mwongozo nurse, faced a common healthcare issue: burnout. He had a demanding schedule with many responsibilities, and the emotional toll of caring for clients weighed heavily on him. Noah had always been the go-to person for help, but he was struggling to cope with mounting stress and exhaustion.

Signs of burnout manifested over time. Noah grew more sceptical about his profession. The tasks that had previously brought him a feeling of fulfilment now seemed burdensome. By the end of each day, he experienced profound emotional exhaustion that lingered well into the night, depriving him of restful sleep.

At first, Noah brushed off his feelings as a fleeting inclination. He pushed himself to his limits, believing that everything would fall into place if he could make it through the upcoming shift and the following week. However, the fatigue persisted, and Noah started to experience a sense of detachment from his work and the individuals under his care. This was a stark departure from the passionate nurse he once was, acknowledged for his compassion and rapport with his clients.

Noah reached his breaking point on a particularly challenging day, marked by complicated client interactions and an overwhelming workload. He found himself in the break room, feeling disheartened. He realised that he could no longer neglect his well-being.

Noah found it challenging to ask for help. He expressed a genuine concern regarding the negative perception surrounding burnout and mental health challenges within the healthcare field. However, realising he was not the only one facing this challenge was a significant turning point. He shared his thoughts with a colleague, who listened attentively and shared her experiences with burnout. This conversation marked the initial stride on Noah's journey toward healing.

Noah started exploring different approaches to managing his stress and workload. He participated in a hospital-sponsored wellness program that offered mindfulness training, stress management courses, and counselling services. These resources equipped Noah with the necessary tools to navigate his emotional exhaustion and prioritise his mental well-being.

He also started advocating for hospital modifications to address nurse burnout. Noah worked closely with hospital administration to develop strategies for reducing workload, enhancing staffing ratios, and offering extra support to nurses. He emerged as an advocate for his colleagues, championing a work environment that acknowledged and addressed nursing concerns.

Noah's adventure also enlightened him about the wonders of breastfeeding. He understood the importance of taking care of oneself personally and professionally. He adjusted his schedule to prioritise breaks, quality time with loved ones, and activities that brought him relaxation and joy.

Noah's perspective on client care transformed as his understanding of the world deepened. He embraced his compassionate and dedicated nurse role, renowned for understanding the importance of balancing caregiving with self-care. His experiences of burnout and recovery brought a fresh perspective to his interactions with clients and coworkers.

Noah's narrative had a profound impact on all individuals at Mercy Mwongozo. His openness regarding his fatigue sparked conversations about mental health and overall wellness among the crew. His endeavours led to tangible changes in the hospital's policy, emphasising the welfare of healthcare providers.

Noah's experience addressing and overcoming burnout within the hospital was compelling. It highlighted a frequently neglected element of carer health and the necessity for institutional changes to support the mental well-being of healthcare professionals. His experience showcased the indomitable spirit of humanity and the profound impact of advocating for mental health in the healthcare sector.

Noah's story went beyond a personal battle; it drove transformation, motivating others to acknowledge and tackle burnout. His journey served as a poignant reminder of the importance of taking care of oneself, not only for the well-being of healthcare providers but also for the level of care they provide to their clients. Noah's story has become integral to Mercy Mwongozo's commitment to fostering a welcoming, nurturing, and sustainable work environment for its staff.

Noah's experience of burnout and subsequent journey of recovery had a profound impact on Mercy Mwongozo Hospital. His openness regarding his challenges encouraged others to share their personal experiences. Sharing ideas and knowledge created a strong bond among the workers, resulting in a nurturing work environment where the welfare of each individual was highly valued.

Noah's advocacy for advancements started to materialise. Hospital administration, appreciating the significance of avoiding burnout, initiated the development of more comprehensive support networks for personnel. These included regular wellness checks, opportunities for professional growth, and efforts to foster a healthy work-life balance.

Noah enthusiastically joined a hospital mentorship program, providing guidance and support to aspiring nurses and healthcare professionals. He shared his insights on stress management, professional boundaries, and the importance of self-care. His insights were invaluable, as they were shaped by a deep understanding and empathy that stemmed from his journey.

Noah's story also led to a series of workshops and seminars at Mercy Mwongozo focusing on resilience in the healthcare field. These seminars provided practical tools and strategies for managing job expectations while highlighting the importance of seeking help.

In addition to his activism, Noah dedicated himself to client care. He ignited discussions about the correlation between the welfare of healthcare personnel and the standard of client care. He advocated for approaches recognising the importance of carer well-being in fulfilling the hospital's mission. This perspective led to a comprehensive approach to healthcare delivery at Mercy Mwongozo, where the well-being of both clients and carers was given equal importance.

In addition, Noah's story sparked a broader conversation about the culture surrounding healthcare. He actively participated in panels and delivered talks both within and outside the hospital, emphasising the necessity of implementing systemic changes to tackle burnout in the healthcare professions. His active participation in these debates brought attention to the issue. It contributed to the creation of policies that placed high importance on the mental well-being of healthcare workers.

Many individuals found inspiration in Noah's transformation from someone who experienced burnout to a passionate advocate for mental health and well-being within the healthcare industry. He had turned a personal challenge into an opportunity to positively impact his company and beyond.

As Noah continued his job, he found a way to prioritise both his work responsibilities and his well-being. He became an exemplary figure in demonstrating how to effectively balance the demands of a healthcare career while maintaining personal well-being.

Noah's experience at Mercy Mwongozo fostered a workplace with increased empathy and a deeper understanding. His experience served as a potent reminder that the well-being of carers is just as important as that of clients. Noah's story has become a significant part of Mercy Mwongozo's culture, symbolising the hospital's commitment to the well-being of its employees and the relentless pursuit of excellence in client care.

Noah's dedication to transforming Mercy Mwongozo Hospital's approach to healthcare worker well-being garnered recognition within the hospital and the broader medical community. His unique approach to addressing burnout was highly praised, serving as a blueprint for other healthcare organisations to emulate.

He collaborated with healthcare organisations and nursing groups, advocating for laws prioritising healthcare professionals' mental and emotional well-being. Through diligent work, he established nationwide protocols for addressing burnout in healthcare environments, emphasising the importance of proactive measures, timely intervention, and robust support systems.

Noah's contributions significantly influenced various aspects of hospital operations at Mercy Mwongozo. Staff turnover rates started to decline, and research indicated a significant improvement in job satisfaction among healthcare personnel. The hospital gained a reputation for its exceptional work environment, drawing in highly skilled individuals and establishing a new standard for employee well-being in the healthcare sector.

Noah also integrated mental health education into hospital staff orientation and ongoing training. These training classes focused on topics like identifying signs of burnout, implementing stress management techniques, and the importance of seeking assistance. By incorporating these elements into the training, Noah successfully fostered a culture within the hospital that prioritised mental health awareness.

In addition, Noah's endeavours led to creating a peer support program at Mercy Mwongozo. This program offered a secure and private space for healthcare professionals to openly discuss their concerns and receive support from colleagues who understood the challenges of the job. The peer support program played a crucial role in dismantling the negative perceptions surrounding mental health, fostering a climate of openness, and encouraging more candid conversations about it.

Noah consistently provides exceptional client care while actively engaging in advocacy efforts. His exhaustion heightened his sensitivity and comprehension, enabling him to better understand and empathise with his clients' needs. He often expressed his perspectives to them, offering guidance and support with a positive and determined attitude as they navigated their paths to better health.

Noah also gained recognition as a sought-after speaker at healthcare conferences and seminars, where he captivated audiences with his compelling story and the strategies he implemented at Mercy

Mwongozo. His thought-provoking presentations inspired fellow healthcare professionals to place a greater emphasis on their mental well-being and advocate for positive transformations in their work environments. He was widely regarded as a symbol of inspiration, demonstrating that overcoming burnout and achieving success in healthcare was feasible.

Noah's contributions at Mercy Mwongozo also positively impacted client care. A more intellectually stimulated workforce led to enhanced client outcomes, increased levels of client satisfaction, and an overall elevation in care quality. The hospital's focus on the well-being of carers became a crucial aspect of its renowned clinical excellence.

Noah's dedication to addressing burnout in healthcare environments grew and developed. He provided crucial information for research projects investigating the long-term impacts of his actions, emphasising the importance of supporting those who provide care. The effect of his work in the healthcare profession is evident, as it redirects the focus toward the welfare of those who dedicate themselves to the care of others.

The narrative of Noah's burnout and subsequent transformation into an advocate for healthcare worker well-being went beyond being a personal experience; it was a driving force for bringing about systemic change. It was a powerful reminder of the human aspect of healthcare, highlighting the significance of a healthcare system that values its professionals as much as its clients. Noah's experience at Mercy Mwongozo showcased the power of resilience, the importance of mental well-being, and a single individual's profound influence in driving transformation in the healthcare field.

Noah's journey became a source of inspiration and resilience for himself and the entire Mercy Mwongozo Hospital community. His wisdom motivated others to confront their challenges bravely and prioritise their welfare. The hospital culture underwent a transformation where vulnerability ceased to be seen as a weakness rather than an inherent aspect of the human condition, particularly in the challenging healthcare field.

This cultural shift had a profound effect on the way employees engaged with each other. There was a noticeable increase in the team's capacity for empathy and understanding. Colleagues tended to keep tabs on each other, assist, or be attentive listeners. This newfound connection fostered a more cohesive and supportive atmosphere in the workplace.

Noah's endeavours also led to a shift towards a healthcare model that prioritises clients' needs. The enhanced welfare of the staff enabled them to engage more deeply with clients, leading to stronger connections and a more empathetic approach to caregiving. This modification was highly appreciated by clients who experienced improved support and care at Mercy Mwongozo.

In addition, Noah's research on burnout garnered positive feedback from healthcare professionals outside of Mercy Mwongozo. The impact of his story and the power of his ideas resonated with other hospitals and healthcare institutions, prompting them to reevaluate their approach to employee well-being. Noah discovered an opportunity to collaborate with a group of healthcare professionals dedicated to creating sustainable work environments that prioritise the mental well-being of healthcare workers.

His advocacy efforts grew, leading him to national and even global platforms where he shared his expertise on preventing burnout. Noah's message highlighted the importance of prioritising the mental well-being of healthcare professionals, not only as a moral obligation but also as a crucial factor in delivering top-notch client care.

Drawn by Noah's work, Mercy Mwongozo's management strongly emphasised their employees' welfare during strategic planning. They implemented policies prioritising a more balanced work-life dynamic, including flexible scheduling and initiatives encouraging employees to take necessary breaks for rejuvenation.

Noah's personal life was shaped by his burnout experience and dedication to enhancing Mercy Mwongozo's work environment. He realised the importance of establishing boundaries, prioritising self-care, and pursuing personal interests beyond work. These enhancements boosted his cognitive well-being and instilled a renewed passion and drive in his career.

Noah observed the fruits of his hard work reflected in the satisfied countenances of his colleagues and the grateful expressions of clients over time. The hospital had become a beacon of hope and an inspiration for other healthcare organisations grappling with staff exhaustion.

Noah's journey of self-discovery and personal growth was a powerful narrative highlighting the importance of mental health support in the healthcare system. The text emphasised the significance of caring for individuals who provide care to others for the benefit of all those involved in the healthcare system. Noah's story at Mercy Mwongozo is an inspiring example of how personal resilience and determination can bring about positive change, enhancing the quality of client care and the lives of carers.

CHAPTER 11

Sophia's Fight for Equity

Sophia, a nurse at Mercy Mwongozo, has always wanted to help underserved communities. Her healthcare career changed significantly when she worked in one of the city's most disadvantaged neighbourhoods. During her exploration, she encountered numerous challenges clients faced, from inadequate access to primary healthcare to societal and economic limitations that hindered their overall welfare. This incident sparked Sophia's unwavering dedication to advocating for equal healthcare access.

Sophia observed the potential consequences of disparities in healthcare access and quality on the lives of individuals in this area. A significant number of her clients had endured prolonged periods without receiving adequate medical care, leading to advanced stages of illnesses that could have been prevented. Sophia was deeply moved by the injustices she witnessed, and she dedicated herself to making a difference by working towards better healthcare accessibility and quality for marginalised communities.

She began by analysing the root causes of these discrepancies. She engaged with individuals in the community, attentively listening to their stories and gaining insights into their experiences with the healthcare system. She earned a valuable understanding of their unique needs and challenges through actively engaging with the community.

Sophia utilised her understanding to develop community outreach programs. She organised health education workshops, free screenings, and immunisation programs. These programs were designed to offer immediate healthcare services and enlighten the population about their health and their rights as clients.

Sophia also collaborated with community organisations to tackle the broader factors that influence health. She understood the significance of housing, nutrition, education, and employment in the community's well-being. Sophia played a crucial role in enhancing community health by working closely with these organisations to develop a more holistic approach.

Her endeavours were worthwhile. Sophia's commitment to the community caught the eye of Mercy Mwongozo's leadership. Appreciating the importance of her work, the hospital offered support and resources to enhance her endeavours. Sophia utilised the funding to broaden her outreach programs and advocate for legislative reforms that positively impact marginalised communities.

Sophia's community work also emphasised the importance of cultural knowledge in healthcare. She educated her colleagues at Mercy Mwongozo on providing considerate and mindful care of their clients' artistic needs. This training fostered more excellent client and provider engagement, cultivating community trust.

Sophia championed the cause of healthcare fairness, tirelessly advocating for those who were unheard. She passionately addressed healthcare forums and public gatherings, shedding light on the pressing issue of healthcare disparities and advocating for comprehensive systemic reform. Her work sheds light on the often-overlooked topics of marginalised areas.

Sophia's work had a profound influence that extended far beyond the local community. She ignited a movement at Mercy Mwongozo and beyond, urging healthcare workers to address healthcare disparities actively. Her example showcased the possibility of achieving change by prioritising understanding and fulfilling all clients' needs, regardless of socioeconomic status.

Sophia's connection with the community deepened as she persisted in her endeavours. She gained widespread recognition for her empathy, unwavering devotion, and belief in equal healthcare access. Her experience showcased an individual's profound impact on transforming the lives of many.

Sophia's story at Mercy Mwongozo and in the underprivileged neighbourhood went beyond a straightforward account of service; it was a powerful depiction of the importance of equal access to healthcare. Her research highlighted the crucial role of healthcare practitioners in advocating for and implementing changes to address gaps in healthcare access and quality. Sophia's experience showcased the power of dedication, compassion, and proactive measures in bringing about significant transformations in the healthcare sector.

Sophia's endeavours started to have a noticeable impact on the community. Her health education courses not only offer essential knowledge but also encourage participants to actively engage in managing their health. Screening and immunisation campaigns have significantly improved access to vital healthcare services, leading to the early detection and control of illnesses.

Her endeavours to tackle the factors influencing health outcomes started showing positive results. Partnerships with local organisations have led to significant nutrition, housing, and education progress. These modifications result in a steady yet evident improvement in the community's well-being.

Sophia was deeply committed to creating a sustainable paradigm for community healthcare. She diligently cultivated partnerships with healthcare providers and organisations to ensure sustained community backing and access to vital resources. These collaborations were essential in guaranteeing that the enhancements were not just temporary fixes but were integral to a lasting transformation in the community's healthcare landscape.

The success of her programs caught the attention of healthcare policymakers. Sophia was invited to participate in healthcare reform debates, where she passionately advocated for legislation that would ensure equal access to healthcare for all populations. Her perspectives, gained from her hands-on experience, were crucial in formulating policies that were more comprehensive and responsive to the needs of marginalised individuals.

Upon her return, Sophia's community experiences influenced Mercy Mwongozo's hospital practices. Her innovative ideas led to progress in nutrition, housing, and education, as well as a client care policy that embraced inclusivity and implemented practices tailored to clients' diverse backgrounds. Drawn by Sophia's work, the hospital personnel became more engaged in community outreach, recognising their crucial role in addressing healthcare inequities.

Sophia was a source of inspiration for other healthcare professionals who were passionate about community health. She imparted her wisdom and insights, inspiring a fresh wave of healthcare professionals committed to fairness and serving their communities. Her guidance fostered a culture of social responsibility within the healthcare profession.

Sophia remained deeply committed to the community as she pursued her work. She was widely recognised for her unwavering dedication and sincere compassion. The trust and respect of the community members were a clear testament to her steadfast commitment and the profound impact of her work.

Sophia's pursuit of healthcare equity was a remarkable tale of empathy, determination, and growth. The text highlighted the profound influence that healthcare professionals can exert when they explore beyond conventional medical environments and address the broader factors that influence health—Sophia's time at Mercy Mwongozo and in the underprivileged community showcased the vital importance of healthcare providers in addressing healthcare inequalities and championing the health and well-being of all individuals.

Sophia's dedication to her community led to expanding her campaign for equitable healthcare. Her programs were sustainable, reproducible, and a model for other communities facing similar challenges. Her approach to community health became a prime example of how to tackle healthcare disparities at the grassroots level.

As healthcare professionals from different locations started visiting Sophia's programs to learn and implement strategies in their communities, a significant impact was experienced. Sophia contributed to these discussions by generously sharing her knowledge and experience. She viewed the pursuit of healthcare equity as a collaborative endeavour that necessitated the exchange of knowledge and cooperation.

Her impact extended to the academic realm as well. Sophia was invited to speak to students at universities and medical schools about the significance of community health and the responsibilities of healthcare professionals in addressing disparities. Her lectures inspired numerous students to pursue careers in community health, thus contributing to the growth of the workforce in this vital healthcare sector.

Sophia actively participated in research initiatives focused on evaluating the effectiveness of different community health programs. The data from these studies provided valuable insights into practical approaches in community health and contributed to creating evidence-based solutions for addressing healthcare disparities.

Sophia's experiences in the community inspired Mercy Mwongozo to adopt a more comprehensive approach to client care. The hospital started incorporating strategies that considered clients' social and economic circumstances. This approach improved client outcomes and satisfaction by considering a more comprehensive range of factors that impact their health.

In addition, Sophia's advocacy activities started to gain recognition on a national scale. She was invited to participate in policy forums and roundtables, where she offered her insights on healthcare equity. Her valuable contributions helped shape policies addressing inequalities and enhancing healthcare access for marginalised individuals.

Sophia's presence in the community was a beacon of hope and motivation. She formed enduring connections with community members, often surpassing her role as a healthcare practitioner to become a trusted advisor and companion. Her unwavering commitment to the community remained strong as she tirelessly advocated for their access to affordable, top-notch healthcare. Sophia's journey showcased the remarkable influence committed healthcare professionals can have on the community's well-being. Her work extended beyond conventional nursing, placing her at the forefront of community health activism.

Sophia's efforts to promote healthcare equity resulted in a more inclusive, compassionate, and effective healthcare system. Her story served as a powerful testament to the transformative impact an individual can have on healthcare and the well-being of countless individuals. Sophia's narrative at Mercy Mwongozo and within the underserved community was an inspiring example and a rallying cry for all healthcare professionals to champion equitable healthcare.

Sophia's unwavering commitment to ensuring equal access to healthcare inspired those around her. Her contributions to Mercy Mwongozo and the community influenced the broader healthcare system. Hospitals and healthcare organisations widely recognised Sophia's strategy as a model for driving significant transformation in delivering healthcare services to underserved regions.

Her steadfast dedication to activism and the impressive achievements of her programs highlighted the pressing importance of healthcare systems being attuned to the socioeconomic circumstances of their clients. This fundamental shift was crucial in tackling the root causes of healthcare inequality.

Sophia played a crucial role in uniting healthcare practitioners, community organisations, and policymakers. These collaborations were pivotal in fostering a unified approach to tackling the intricate issues surrounding healthcare disparity. She believed that achieving lasting change required the cooperation of all parties involved in healthcare delivery.

Sophia consistently provided guidance and support to her colleagues at Mercy Mwongozo. She encouraged them to take the initiative in community health and consider the broader context of their client's lives when developing care plans. Her impact was instrumental in shaping a new breed of healthcare professionals who excelled in their medical expertise and unwavering dedication to their clients.

Sophia's work also led to the development of community-based health programs tailored to meet the needs of different groups.

These programs focused on promoting preventive care, educating about health, and intervening early, leading to a significant decrease in the prevalence of avoidable illnesses among the population.

Her efforts significantly improved the health outcomes and quality of life in the communities she served. In these communities, previously overlooked by the healthcare system, residents now have enhanced access to healthcare and a deeper understanding of prioritising their well-being.

Sophia's journey and her improvements were a powerful demonstration of the potential of empathetic, community-centred healthcare. Her story went beyond triumph over challenges; it transformed the healthcare landscape towards equality and fairness.

Sophia remained intricately connected to the individuals she served as she continued her work. She was widely recognised and highly regarded for her unwavering dedication to improving the lives of those in her community. Her narrative of advocating for healthcare equity at Mercy Mwongozo and in underserved communities showcased the profound influence of committed healthcare professionals. The importance of acknowledging clients' diverse needs and the crucial role of healthcare providers in addressing disparities in healthcare access and quality was underscored. Sophia's experience showcased the power of commitment, compassion, and teamwork in driving significant progress in public health and fostering a fairer healthcare system.

CHAPTER 12

The Digital Conundrum

Emma, a nurse at Mercy Mwongozo Hospital, was at the forefront of a new era in healthcare: the emergence of telemedicine. Emma fully embraced the transformative power of digital technologies in revolutionising medical care, understanding their ability to enhance client accessibility and convenience. However, she soon faced a dilemma that challenged her beliefs about the essence of client care.

Emma's transition to telehealth was seamless. She was amazed by the effectiveness and global reach of Internet consultations, which enabled her to connect with clients who would otherwise have been unable to access healthcare. As she delved further into this unfamiliar realm of healthcare, Emma started to feel a sense of detachment. The screens and technologies that facilitated these encounters also appeared to create an unforeseen obstacle.

Emma failed to appreciate the nuances of in-person care, including the opportunity to interact with a client physically, interpret subtle cues from their body language, and establish a personal bond that can only be forged in the same physical space. She believed a crucial element of the healing process had been overlooked during the shift from physical to digital connections.

Driven by her curiosity, Emma embarked on a quest to explore methods of infusing telehealth meetings with a sense of warmth and personal connection. She experimented with various video conversation methods, emphasising the importance of conveying emotions and dedicating additional time to address her clients' concerns attentively. She aimed to ensure that every telemedicine session was as personal and captivating as an in-person appointment.

Emma initiated conversations with her colleagues and hospital administration about the constraints of telehealth. She emphasised the need for training programs to support healthcare professionals in enhancing their communication skills in a digital environment. Through her endeavours, she successfully developed seminars that focus on fostering empathy and encouraging the active involvement of clients in telehealth environments.

Appreciating the importance of client feedback, Emma proactively sought input from her clients regarding their telehealth experiences. This feedback was crucial in comprehending the clients' perspectives and implementing the necessary adjustments to enhance the digital healthcare experience.

Her hard work started to yield results. Clients expressed higher satisfaction with their telehealth appointments, highlighting the sincere care and connection they experienced during virtual encounters. Emma's flexibility influenced the quality of care she could provide digitally.

Despite these advancements, Emma found herself faced with the limitations of telehealth. She acknowledged that some aspects of client care, especially physical examinations and procedures, could not be replicated digitally. She worked with the hospital to develop a unique approach to client care, combining telemedicine for follow-ups and consultations with in-person appointments for more comprehensive examinations and treatments.

Emma's digital dilemma highlighted the challenge of integrating technology into healthcare. It emphasised the importance of maintaining a personal connection in medicine, particularly in a world increasingly reliant on technology. Her time at Mercy Mwongozo was marked by adaptability, ingenuity, and an unwavering commitment to providing compassionate in-person or virtual care.

Emma's telehealth experiences encompassed more than adapting to a novel approach to healthcare provision. They involved finding a harmonious equilibrium between the effectiveness of technology and the essential human connection that lies at the core of client care. Her journey provided a thought-provoking glimpse into the evolving landscape of digital healthcare and the importance of placing the human factor at the forefront of medical care.

Emma's exploration into telehealth started to impact the overall protocols at Mercy Mwongozo Hospital. Her insightful input and constructive feedback played a pivotal role in shaping the hospital's approach to digital healthcare. She advocated for a telemedicine strategy focused on putting clients first, emphasising empathy, and fostering meaningful connections rather than solely prioritising efficiency.

Her work focused on developing telehealth standards, highlighting the importance of effective communication, active client involvement, and empathetic presence. These principles helped other healthcare providers quickly adjust to the digital environment, ensuring that clients felt valued and well-attended, even through a screen.

Emma embarked on community outreach programs driven by the recognition of telehealth's ability to address disparities in healthcare access. She collaborated with local organisations to introduce telehealth services to underdeveloped areas, ensuring disadvantaged populations access top-notch healthcare. This project significantly impacted rural areas, where citizens often faced challenges in accessing medical services.

Emma played a crucial role in coordinating virtual health education seminars. These events facilitated the exchange of essential knowledge regarding various health issues and fostered engaging conversations between healthcare professionals and community members. The success of these sessions showcased the immense potential of telehealth in promoting community education and engagement.

Emma's experience with telehealth has sparked curiosity in research on the effectiveness of digital healthcare. She collaborated with research teams to explore client outcomes, satisfaction, and the efficiency of telehealth services. The findings of this study provided valuable insights into the strengths and limitations of digital healthcare, which will guide future advancements and developments.

Emma became a valuable asset for colleagues transitioning to telehealth at Mercy Mwongozo, providing her insights and recommendations for effective digital interactions. Her expertise helped numerous healthcare providers navigate the intricacies of virtual client care with increased assurance and proficiency.

Emma deeply understood the importance of building personal connections in healthcare as she integrated telehealth into her business. She started incorporating small yet significant practices into her telemedicine sessions, like taking a few minutes at the beginning of each call to have personal conversations with her clients. This approach facilitated the establishment of a strong connection and confidence, which contributed to the clients' increased comfort.

Her efforts to bring a more human touch to digital healthcare were not in vain. Clients often expressed appreciation for the sense of care and attention they felt during virtual encounters. Clients' reactions were overwhelmingly positive, validating Emma's efforts to incorporate empathy and compassion into telehealth.

Emma's impact was felt in discussions on telehealth policy at both regional and national levels. She championed legislation that promoted the integration of telehealth into standard healthcare practices, guaranteeing that digital healthcare services were available, fair, and focused on clients' needs.

Emma's digital challenge became a chance for personal development and unleashing her creative potential. Her story exemplified how healthcare workers can successfully navigate and embrace digital technology advancements while prioritising emotional connection in client care.

Her journey also highlighted the importance of being adaptable and flexible in healthcare. Emma showcased the importance of being versatile and innovative to effectively engage with and care for clients in a rapidly evolving medical landscape.

Emma's experience at Mercy Mwongozo Hospital unfolded as a tale of triumph over the constraints of contemporary healthcare. It was a narrative that explored the integration of technology with timeless values like empathy and compassion, emphasising the importance of preserving the human element in an increasingly digital healthcare landscape.

Emma's journey into telehealth continued to grow as she explored innovative technology and methods to enhance client care. Her work in this field showcased healthcare professionals' adaptability, resilience, and capacity to solve emerging challenges creatively.

Emma's story in the world of digital healthcare highlighted the importance of personal connection in the healing process.

Emma's telehealth experience significantly shaped the future of digital healthcare at Mercy Mwongozo Hospital. She collaborated with the information technology department to enhance the telehealth platform, ensuring its ease of use and accessibility for clients of all ages. Her contribution was crucial in developing a user-friendly interface and reducing the technological barriers that often deter clients from utilising telehealth services.

She has also started focusing on teaching healthcare practitioners the art of digital communication. Emma coordinated workshops that delved into the technical and human aspects of telehealth. She showcased her ability to maintain eye contact while filming, analyse client expressions and body language, and express empathy and understanding in a virtual scenario. This training helped healthcare providers enhance their ability to provide clients with a more engaging and comforting telehealth experience.

Emma's endeavours beyond the hospital encompassed reaching out to the broader community. She understood that the success of telehealth relied not only on healthcare providers but also on client acceptance and adaptability. Emma initiated community education programs to make telehealth more accessible, educate individuals on digital healthcare services, and dispel common concerns and misunderstandings.

Emma's dedication to improving telehealth services drove her to explore the lasting effects of digital healthcare delivery. She actively engaged in studies examining client health outcomes, satisfaction levels, and the effectiveness of telemedicine in managing chronic diseases. The findings of this study were crucial in refining telehealth methods and ensuring that digital healthcare services effectively complement traditional in-person care.

Her encounter with telehealth showcased the immense potential of digital technology in revolutionising healthcare delivery. Emma passionately championed using telehealth for various purposes, including regular check-ups, mental well-being support, and health education. The increased utilisation of telehealth services has a significant impact on enhancing the accessibility and effectiveness of healthcare.

Emma was a strong advocate for integrating telehealth into emergency medicine. She dedicated her efforts to developing protocols that enabled rapid virtual consultations during emergencies, ensuring clients in critical conditions received prompt guidance and assistance. This innovative approach to emergency care showcases the adaptability and possibilities of telehealth in different medical scenarios.

Emma's telehealth work had a far-reaching impact beyond the medical field. Her efforts contributed to a greater understanding of the importance of digital healthcare in today's medical field. Other healthcare facilities started to view Mercy Mwongozo as a benchmark for effectively integrating telehealth services.

Emma's encounter with telehealth unfolded as a captivating tale of healthcare ingenuity and flexibility. When applied with wisdom and empathy, the example showcased the positive impact of using digital technology to enhance healthcare. Her example highlighted the importance of adapting to new circumstances while upholding fundamental principles of client care.

Emma was committed to upholding the human aspect of healthcare as she delved into the potential of telehealth. Her experience at

Mercy Mwongozo Hospital went beyond adapting to a new healthcare approach. It involved leading the charge toward a future where technology and human interaction harmoniously blend, leading to a healthcare system that is more accessible, efficient, and empathetic. Emma's narrative in digital healthcare served as a guiding light, illuminating a future where technology enhances, rather than supplants, the fundamental human elements of healthcare.

Emma's efforts to incorporate telemedicine into standard healthcare practices have become crucial to client care at Mercy Mwongozo Hospital. Her unwavering commitment to enhancing the telehealth experience led to the creation of groundbreaking inventions that revolutionised virtual client-provider interactions.

One notable innovation was creating a virtual waiting room, where clients could access information about their illness, familiarise themselves with the hospital's services, and prepare for their visit in a pleasant and informative environment. This feature improved the telehealth experience by eliminating the impersonal nature often associated with online consultations.

Emma played a crucial role in integrating telemedicine into chronic disease management programs. She created a system that allowed clients to meet regularly with their healthcare providers to receive immediate guidance on medication, lifestyle adjustments, and techniques for managing their illnesses. This method proved particularly beneficial for individuals with limited mobility or residing in remote areas.

Emma also understood the importance of feedback in enhancing telehealth services. She implemented a system that enabled clients to quickly provide feedback on their telehealth experience. This feedback was crucial in ensuring the service aligned with the client's needs and expectations and was consistently enhanced.

Emma thoroughly explored the application of augmented reality (AR) and virtual reality (VR) technology in her mission to make telemedicine more personable. She envisioned a future where these technologies would be harnessed to cultivate increasingly immersive and interactive healthcare experiences, seamlessly bridging the realms of physical and digital healthcare.

She demonstrated a deep understanding and appreciation for the potential of telehealth, extending its benefits beyond just client care. Emma understood the importance of safeguarding data security and privacy in the digital realm. She worked closely with the hospital's information technology department to ensure the safety and compliance of all telehealth contacts with healthcare privacy rules. The focus on privacy and security has significantly built trust between clients and providers regarding telehealth services.

Emma's telemedicine initiatives ignited a surge of awareness and investment in digital healthcare technologies at Mercy Mwongozo. The hospital started to gain recognition as a trailblazer in innovative client care solutions, attracting attention from healthcare providers and organisations around the globe.

Emma's telemedicine journey inspired other healthcare professionals. She emphasised the importance of creativity, compassion, and a client-focused mindset in transforming the challenges of telemedicine into opportunities to enhance healthcare provision.

Her experience at Mercy Mwongozo Hospital evolved into pursuing innovation and leading the way to enhance client care. The focus was on finding a harmonious blend of technological advancement and the essential human element that sets healthcare apart. Emma's narrative in digital healthcare remains a source of inspiration and guidance, shaping a future where technology is harnessed to enhance and nurture the bond between clients and carers, going beyond mere convenience.

CHAPTER 13

Global Outreach

A nurse at Mercy Mwongozo Hospital, David has always been captivated by global health. His journey took a significant turn when he immersed himself in global nursing initiatives, which allowed him to contribute his expertise to different countries and tackle the pressing health challenges marginalised communities face.

His initial endeavour occurred in a rural African village with a dire need for primary healthcare. David quickly noticed that the healthcare infrastructure and resources significantly differed from what he was accustomed to at Mercy Mwongozo. This experience gave him a firsthand understanding of the challenges in global health and the importance of providing culturally sensitive care.

David worked closely with local healthcare personnel in this community, exchanging knowledge and expertise. He implemented essential healthcare practices and trained community health workers, emphasising preventive care and primary treatment for common ailments. This cooperative approach helped enhance the community's immediate healthcare needs and empowered the local healthcare staff.

David's involvement in these global endeavours expanded his perspectives on his nursing career. He developed a knack for being resourceful, often finding creative solutions with limited resources to provide the highest-quality care. Through these experiences, he gained a deeper understanding of global health disparities and the impact of socioeconomic factors on health.

His work had a profound influence. The populations he served experienced a significant enhancement in healthcare awareness and outcomes. David's commitment to working with local healthcare practitioners ensured that the changes would have a lasting impact even after his projects were finished.

David returned to Mercy Mwongozo and shared his experiences and lessons with his coworkers. He orchestrated workshops and seminars to emphasise worldwide health issues and possibilities. His stories and observations inspired numerous Mercy Mwongozo employees to contemplate participating in global health programs.

David was crucial in establishing partnerships between Mercy Mwongozo and healthcare organisations worldwide. These collaborations emphasised exchange programs where healthcare workers from Mercy Mwongozo could participate in global health projects, and professionals from other countries could visit Mercy Mwongozo to learn and exchange their expertise.

David's extensive international experiences have influenced his passionate advocacy for incorporating global health education into nursing courses. He worked closely with educational institutions to integrate global health topics into the curriculum, preparing future nurses for a healthcare landscape that is becoming more interconnected.

He also ventured into policy formulation for international healthcare efforts as part of his global health journey. He brought knowledge to the table, passionately advocating for policies prioritising healthcare's long-term development in underserved areas.

A strong commitment, a thirst for knowledge, and a significant influence characterised David's experience at Mercy Mwongozo and in his overseas work. The focus was bridging boundaries to tackle worldwide healthcare issues and sharing knowledge and skills to enhance global health results. His journey showcased nurses' significant impact on global health, working towards a future where quality healthcare is accessible to everyone.

David's participation in international nursing endeavours and his impact on global health expanded. Every project he undertook broadened his understanding of various healthcare systems and the unique challenges different communities face. He served as a bridge between continents, facilitating the exchange of resources, knowledge, and people.

He dedicated a significant amount of his time and energy to South America, specifically working on community health education to combat the transmission of contagious diseases. David's approach here extended beyond disease treatment; he aimed to enlighten the community about preventive hygiene and good living practices. Through his diligent work, he successfully decreased the occurrence of avoidable illnesses in the regions to which he dedicated himself.

David's experiences at Mercy Mwongozo significantly impacted hospital practices related to global health engagements. He passionately advocated for Mercy Mwongozo to transform into a worldwide health excellence centre where healthcare professionals would receive comprehensive training in clinical skills and global health complexities. As a result, a global health department was established, focusing on developing programs and partnerships for international health initiatives.

David also took on the role of mentoring nurses interested in pursuing careers in global health. He generously imparted his wisdom and insights to them, guiding them through the intricacies and rewards of working in diverse healthcare environments. His expertise helped shape a new wave of nurses with a global perspective and a deep understanding of different cultures.

David's efforts extended worldwide, encompassing humanitarian aid in times of crisis. He participated in medical missions following natural disasters, providing essential care in challenging circumstances. His capacity to adjust and provide assistance in these difficult circumstances showcased his skills and commitment.

His passion for global health led him to collaborate on public health initiatives with international organisations. These campaigns focused on essential topics such as immunisation, maternal health, and disease prevention, effectively reaching a broad audience and significantly contributing to global public health outcomes.

David's work profoundly affected the well-being of the communities he served and raised awareness of global health issues among his colleagues and the broader medical community. His journey sparked a newfound motivation and a rallying cry for healthcare professionals to engage in global health.

David's story at Mercy Mwongozo and his overseas work exemplified the profound impact healthcare professionals can have in creating a more equitable and healthier world. His journey showcased the power of dedication, empathy, and a willingness to acquire knowledge and adjust, resulting in substantial improvements in global health. David's story remains a source of inspiration and motivation, emphasising the importance of a broad outlook and teamwork in the dynamic healthcare field.

David's international healthcare activities became a prime example of successful global nursing practice. His unique approach to integrating clinical expertise, cultural awareness, and community involvement became a hallmark of his work, influencing how global health initiatives were approached and executed.

During one of his Southeast Asian projects, David deeply integrated traditional health practices with modern treatment methods. He worked closely with native healers, gaining knowledge about their practices and incorporating their valuable insights into healthcare programs. This holistic approach enhanced the treatment experience and fostered a sense of camaraderie, admiration, and confidence within the community.

Drawn by David's work, Mercy Mwongozo's global health department initiated a nurse exchange program. This program enabled Mercy Mwongozo nurses to gain experience in international settings while allowing nurses from different countries to come to Mercy Mwongozo and exchange knowledge. The exchange program was a highly enriching experience for all participants, broadening horizons and fostering a greater understanding of global health.

David also developed a keen interest in research projects that tackle global health issues. He collaborated with international health organisations to research effective disease control techniques, the influence of cultural practices on health, and the creation of healthcare models for resource-limited settings. The research findings provided valuable insights and contributed to the global knowledge base on effective healthcare procedures.

Furthermore, David's unwavering commitment to advancing global health education led him to develop online courses and webinars. By utilising these digital platforms, he was able to disseminate his knowledge and insights to a broader audience, connecting with healthcare professionals and students worldwide. He offered courses covering global health ethics and disease-specific treatment techniques in resource-constrained situations.

David's campaign for global health also involved active engagement in developing international policies. He was invited to participate in global health policy talks, where he contributed his practical knowledge and thoughts to the discussion. His contributions helped shape policies grounded in healthcare delivery's practicalities across different scenarios.

David's mere presence brought a sense of optimism and achievement to the places he worked. He provided healthcare and encouraged individuals to assume responsibility for their well-being. He educated local healthcare personnel, established community health committees, and implemented health education programs to empower communities with the necessary knowledge and skills to sustain their health advancements.

David's journey in global health was a continuous source of knowledge and growth. He had a keen appetite for fresh ideas and approaches, constantly adapting his strategies to address the dynamic challenges of healthcare delivery across different scenarios. His work showcased the belief that effective care necessitates a blend of scientific expertise, empathy, and cultural understanding.

The story of David's global outreach at Mercy Mwongozo and beyond unfolded as a testament to innovation, commitment, and collaboration across different cultures. The text highlighted the crucial role of nurses in global health and their significant contribution to enhancing health outcomes and advocating for healthcare equity. David's experience exemplified the power of dedication and a broad worldview in driving transformative advancements in the healthcare industry.

His work ignited inspiration and motivation among his colleagues at Mercy Mwongozo and across the globe. David's story was a personal triumph and a testament to the power of passion, expertise, and a profound understanding of cultural intricacies in advancing a more equitable and efficient global healthcare system. His journey was a powerful reminder of the vital role that healthcare professionals play in addressing healthcare disparities and improving global health.

David's efforts in global health gained widespread recognition, profoundly impacting the communities he served and the healthcare community as a whole. His approach, which integrates practical care with thoughtful planning and collaboration, set a new standard for global nursing initiatives.

Appreciating the importance of long-term health initiatives in the communities he worked with, David focused on developing them. He was crucial in setting up local health clinics, ensuring they had the necessary resources and personnel to provide continuous care. These clinics have proven essential health services, offering convenient and ongoing treatment while reducing the burden of clients travelling long distances for medical care.

His research in these fields highlighted the importance of proactive healthcare. David orchestrated extensive vaccination campaigns and routine health check-ups, which played a crucial role in averting outbreaks of infectious diseases. These proactive measures improved the community's well-being and laid the foundation for a more promising future.

David's experiences abroad impacted healthcare policy significantly, as did his hands-on initiatives. He pursued a career as a consultant for international health organisations, guiding the implementation of impactful and culturally sensitive healthcare initiatives. His practical and experience-driven perspectives played a crucial role in shaping global health strategies and policies.

David's diverse global experiences enhanced Mercy Mwongozo Hospital's approach to healthcare. He brought back innovative ideas and practices incorporated into the hospital's operations, improving client care and expanding the range of services offered.

David played a crucial role in fostering a culture of global health awareness among his coworkers. He regularly held debriefing sessions where he openly discussed his experiences, challenges, and successes from his international work. These workshops educated and motivated his colleagues to delve into their contributions to global health.

David's active participation in international health initiatives has led to establishing a prestigious global health fellowship program at Mercy Mwongozo. This program allows healthcare professionals to work internationally, making valuable contributions to global health initiatives and gaining practical experience.

David's contributions made a significant impact in the academic world as well. He collaborated with institutions to develop case studies inspired by his international journeys. These case studies are essential learning resources for healthcare students, offering real-world examples of global health issues and solutions.

David's pursuit of global health continued to expand as he explored fresh strategies for tackling the dynamic landscape of global healthcare needs. His unwavering commitment to achieving fairness in worldwide health and exceptional adaptability in navigating diverse healthcare scenarios earned him widespread admiration within the profession.

The narrative of David's global health work at Mercy Mwongozo and beyond showcased the power of empathy, cultural awareness, and teamwork in tackling global healthcare challenges. His story remains a source of inspiration and guidance, showcasing the profound impact healthcare professionals can have on the world, one community at a time.

CHAPTER 14

Revolutionising Education

Lina, a nurse educator at Mercy Mwongozo Hospital, embarked on a mission to revolutionise how nursing was taught. Her passion for learning and her conviction in the power of creative teaching methods motivated her to explore new frontiers in nursing education. Lina saw the limitations of the traditional lecture-based approach and sought to create a more interactive, captivating, and fruitful learning atmosphere for her students.

She began incorporating technology into her classroom instruction. Lina integrated virtual simulations and interactive software into the curriculum, allowing students to enhance their skills in lifelike scenarios. This interactive approach motivated students to learn through active participation, enhancing the learning experience with a sense of engagement and lasting impact.

Lina understood the importance of interprofessional education in nursing. She collaborated with various departments to coordinate integrated classes, allowing nursing students to gain knowledge alongside their peers in medicine, pharmacy, and social work. These interdisciplinary seminars enhanced the understanding of client care for future healthcare providers and fostered a sense of teamwork and collaboration.

Lina fully embraced the concept of flipped classrooms in her pursuit of innovative teaching methods. She offered students reading and lecture materials to review outside class and dedicated class time to engage in debates, hands-on activities, and group projects. This approach fostered a culture of critical thinking and empowered students to delve further into the subject matter.

Lina's innovative methods went beyond the confines of the classroom. She facilitated opportunities for students to engage in practical, hands-on learning experiences within the community. These experiences were precious as they exposed students to diverse client care scenarios and aided in their understanding of the broader social and environmental factors that impact health.

Lina also highlighted the importance of soft skills in nursing education. She integrated modules focused on effective communication, understanding others' perspectives, and guiding a team into the program. These skills were essential in teaching students to become empathetic carers, accomplished leaders in healthcare settings, and proficient nurses.

Lina's efforts to transform nursing education started to gain momentum. Her techniques enhanced student involvement and long-term understanding. Her students' feedback was overwhelmingly positive, with many expressing that her classes were a pivotal experience in their education.

Her endeavours also caught the interest of the broader educational community. Lina has been invited to speak at conferences and workshops, where she has shared her innovative techniques and motivated other educators to reevaluate their teaching practices. Her influence expanded, shaping the progress of nursing education.

Lina consistently explores and embraces new teaching tactics, ensuring she remains current on the latest educational trends and innovations. Her commitment to groundbreaking teaching methods revolutionised nursing education at Mercy Mwongozo and beyond, solidifying her reputation as a trailblazer in the field.

Lina's story of revolutionising nursing education was a testament to her innovative thinking, unwavering dedication, and contagious passion. It revolved around challenging the status quo and embracing innovative approaches to education. Lina's journey showcased the power of forward-thinking educational methods in enhancing learning experiences and equipping students with the necessary skills to navigate contemporary healthcare challenges.

Lina's innovative teaching methods enhanced the educational environment at Mercy Mwongozo Hospital. Her unique approach resonated with students and teachers, igniting a previously unexplored passion for education and a newfound excitement for nursing.

Lina primarily focused on implementing learning experiences and prioritising clients' needs and preferences. She facilitated opportunities for nursing students to engage with clients, allowing them to gain valuable insights from their experiences and perspectives. This approach enhanced the students' clinical skills and expanded their comprehension of client care from a holistic standpoint.

Lina was also a pioneer in using client narratives as a teaching technique. She encouraged clients to share their experiences with the students, offering valuable perspectives on their journey through the healthcare system. These stories helped students understand the importance of their role and the value of compassion and empathy in nursing practice.

Lina also highlighted the importance of fostering critical thinking and problem-solving skills among her students. She presented them with thought-provoking case studies and fostered a collaborative environment where they could work together to create care plans and take action. This problem-solving approach empowered students to tackle real-world challenges in healthcare settings.

Her commitment to education extended beyond the classroom and medical facility confines. Lina collaborated with online learning platforms to develop nursing courses that a more comprehensive range of learners could easily access. These courses covered various subjects, from fundamental nursing skills to advanced clinical procedures, providing aspiring nurses worldwide with greater access to high-quality nursing education.

Lina's impact can also be observed in her advocacy for ongoing professional development for registered nurses. She emphasised the importance of continuous learning in nursing. Mercy Mwongozo Hospital started organising regular workshops, seminars, and training sessions for its nursing staff under her guidance, ensuring that they stayed informed about the most recent methods and advancements in healthcare.

Lina's teaching methods had a profound influence. The nursing students who were trained under her guidance became well-informed, empathetic, and creative professionals who were equipped to tackle the challenges of contemporary healthcare. They possessed the knowledge and skills that Lina had imparted to them and the principles and morals that Lina had ingrained in them.

Lina's experience at Mercy Mwongozo Hospital became a captivating tale of transforming nursing education through ingenuity, originality, and an unwavering commitment to student success. Her journey exemplified the transformative power of education in shaping healthcare professionals and, consequently, enhancing the standard of client care. Lina's forward-thinking teaching methods continue to inspire and make a lasting impact on the future of nursing education, emphasising educators' crucial role in shaping the healthcare professionals of tomorrow.

Lina's efforts to transform nursing education at Mercy Mwongozo Hospital garnered significant recognition. Her techniques were widely acknowledged for their effectiveness, prompting other institutions to seek her expertise. Lina was excited to share her knowledge, passionately believing in the potential of collaboration to enhance nursing education globally.

She embarked on speaking engagements at nursing schools and healthcare conferences. During these sessions, Lina highlighted the importance of adapting nursing education to align with the evolving demands of the healthcare industry. She showcased the potential of interactive learning, seamless integration of technology, and a client-centred approach to enhance the educational experience and equip students with the skills needed to tackle real-world nursing challenges.

Lina also developed a keen interest in studying nursing educational approaches. She collaborated with scholars to explore the impacts of different teaching approaches, presenting compelling evidence that affirmed the value of engaging and immersive academic encounters. Her research played a significant role in shaping evidence-based practices in nursing education, profoundly impacting the curriculum development at multiple nursing schools.

Lina's dedication also led to establishing a mentorship program at Mercy Mwongozo. This program paired seasoned nurses with nursing students and recent graduates to offer mentorship, assistance, and real-world perspectives on the nursing field. The mentorship program was a resounding success, effectively connecting theory and practice.

Lina's commitment to advancing nursing education is evident in her incorporation of global health concepts into the curriculum. She coordinated international exchange programs that provided students and professors with valuable exposure to diverse healthcare systems and nursing practices from across the globe. These experiences expanded students' knowledge of global health issues and the impact of nurses on addressing them.

Lina played a significant role in the development of community engagement programs. She encouraged her students to actively participate in community health initiatives that offer care and education in disadvantaged communities. These programs not only had a positive impact on the communities, but they also provided students with valuable hands-on learning experiences.

Lina's educational pursuits yielded fruitful collaborations with technology companies focused on healthcare. These collaborations created new simulation technologies and e-learning resources, enriching the learning experience for nursing students.

Lina's reputation soared, yet she remained steadfast in her unwavering belief that the goal of nursing school was to cultivate empathetic, skilled, and tenacious healthcare professionals. She consistently pursued new approaches to enhance the learning experience and equip her students for the dynamic healthcare industry.

Lina's journey at Mercy Mwongozo transformed into a catalyst for revolutionising nursing education. The story revolves around exploring uncharted territory, embracing new ideas, and relentlessly striving for excellence in nursing education for future generations. Her experience showcased the profound influence that a committed educator can wield in shaping the future of a profession. Lina's innovative teaching methods continue to inspire and impact nursing education, highlighting educators' crucial role in fostering growth and excellence in the healthcare field.

Lina's innovative approach to nursing education revolutionised the curriculum at Mercy Mwongozo Hospital and the institution's learning culture. Her creative strategies sparked students' renewed curiosity and enthusiasm for nursing, fostering a vibrant, interactive, and highly stimulating learning atmosphere.

Her impact reached far and wide, shaping the methods of clinical training. Lina introduced scenario-based training sessions where students can practice high-pressure situations in a secure environment. This approach not only enhanced their clinical skills but also provided them with emotional and mental readiness for the challenges of the nursing profession.

Lina incorporated stress management and self-care into the curriculum, acknowledging the significance of emotional resilience in nursing. She conducted workshops and seminars to educate students on maintaining their well-being while managing the demands of their profession. These sessions were essential in equipping students to handle the emotional challenges of nursing. Lina's approach dramatically influences the academic achievements and self-assurance of her students. They completed their nursing education, demonstrating proficiency in their field. Additionally, they developed emotional intelligence and adaptability, preparing them to take on leadership positions in the healthcare industry.

Lina's hard work also led to establishing a community of practice among nursing educators. She created platforms and communities for educators to share their thoughts, difficulties, and achievements. This group has developed into a platform for ongoing learning and growth in nursing education, cultivating an innovative and exceptional culture.

Lina's work also caught the interest of healthcare policymakers and leaders. She was invited to participate in national discussions on healthcare education, where she advocated for nursing education reforms that align more effectively with current healthcare needs. Her astute observations were pivotal in influencing policies in nursing education, prioritising the development of practical skills, emotional intelligence, and adaptability. Lina remained dedicated to her vision of enhancing nursing education as she persisted in her efforts. She consistently kept up with the latest trends and technologies in healthcare and education, continuously adapting her approaches to ensure they stayed up-to-date and impactful.

Lina's work at Mercy Mwongozo Hospital exemplified the impact of forward-thinking and determination in bringing about meaningful transformation in nursing education. It highlighted educators' crucial impact on shaping healthcare professionals' future. Lina's journey and innovative teaching methods have had a lasting effect, showcasing the significance of education in cultivating skilled, empathetic, and adaptable healthcare professionals.

CHAPTER 15

Voice for the Voiceless

Aisha, a nurse at Mercy Mwongozo Hospital, has always understood the importance of cultural competence in healthcare. She embarked on a journey driven by a keen observation: people from diverse backgrounds often faced obstacles when accessing healthcare. These clients encountered various challenges, including language barriers, cultural misconceptions, and a shortage of healthcare providers who understood their unique needs. Aisha saw this as a question of fairness and equality, not just a healthcare service.

Aisha embarked on a mission to foster cultural understanding at Mercy Mwongozo, unwavering in her commitment to advocate for those whose voices often go unheard. She began by organising a series of workshops and seminars for hospital employees. These workshops were designed to educate and raise awareness among healthcare providers about different cultural beliefs and practices and how they can influence healthcare.

Aisha's endeavours extended beyond education. She advocated for the hospital to expand its staff diversity, recognising the potential for a more compassionate and efficient healthcare team. Her hard work paid off when the hospital administration changed to promote a more inclusive employment process.

Aisha recognised the significance of language in client care and took the initiative to implement a program providing language interpretation services within the hospital. This program was a significant advancement in bridging the communication divide between healthcare providers and clients who speak multiple languages. It ensured all clients received clear and understandable information about their health and treatment choices.

Her endeavours extended beyond the institution's boundaries. Aisha collaborated with community leaders and organisations to better understand and address the diverse health needs within the hospital's catchment area. She orchestrated community health fairs that were mindful of cultural sensitivities, providing individuals with health tests, information, and resources.

In addition, Aisha's hard work led to creating a client advisory board at Mercy Mwongozo. This board, comprised of individuals from diverse backgrounds, offered valuable insights and recommendations on how the hospital could improve its services and foster inclusivity.

Aisha's endeavours had a profound impact. Clients from various backgrounds started to show increased satisfaction with the care they received at Mercy Mwongozo. By fostering a deeper understanding and providing ample resources to address cultural differences, the staff was able to deliver treatment that was both respectful and effective.

As her work advanced, Aisha gained recognition in cultural competency in healthcare. She has been invited to speak at conferences and panels, where she has shared her insights and strategies for enhancing healthcare delivery in different regions.

Aisha's work at Mercy Mwongozo Hospital is a compelling testament to a committed individual's profound influence in transforming healthcare norms. Her narrative showcased the significance of a deep understanding of different cultures in the healthcare field and the crucial role of speaking up for those often overlooked. Aisha's tireless dedication continued to inspire and guide, leading the way toward a healthcare environment characterised by respect, inclusivity, and equity for everyone.

Aisha's efforts at Mercy Mwongozo Hospital to promote cultural competency started to make a noticeable difference in the broader healthcare community. The success of her programs emphasised the tangible advantages of understanding and valuing cultural diversity in healthcare environments. Mercy Mwongozo has become a shining example of cultural competency for other hospitals and healthcare facilities.

Aisha's commitment to this cause led her to develop a comprehensive cultural competence training curriculum incorporated into Mercy Mwongozo's ongoing education for all staff. The program covered cultural sensitivity, effective communication strategies, and the impact of cultural beliefs on health and healthcare decisions. This training was essential to the hospital's dedication to delivering care and prioritising client needs.

Aisha highlighted the importance of involving clients and their families in the care process to promote inclusivity in healthcare. She emphasised the importance of healthcare providers engaging in open and respectful interactions with clients, considering their cultural values and preferences when developing care plans.

Aisha's efforts focused on expanding healthcare access for marginalised communities. She dedicated her efforts to outreach programs targeting these populations, providing healthcare directly to their homes. These programs provided essential medical care, facilitated the establishment of trust, and eliminated barriers between healthcare providers and the community.

Aisha's diligent work also positively influenced the clients' outcomes. Clients from diverse backgrounds experienced significant improvements in their health as they received tailored care that met their specific needs. The hospital has made tremendous progress in reducing health disparities, moving closer to its goal of providing fair and equal healthcare to everyone.

In addition, Aisha's dedication to promoting cultural understanding led to significant policy changes at both the regional and national levels. She was invited to participate in policy talks, where her insights contributed to developing more culturally sensitive and inclusive healthcare policies.

Aisha was deeply committed to promoting cultural competence throughout her career. She stayed well-informed about the latest research and advancements in the field, ensuring that her work was always grounded in the most reliable evidence.

Aisha's endeavours at Mercy Mwongozo Hospital unfolded as a compelling tale of transformation and advancement in the healthcare industry. Understanding and valuing cultural differences in enhancing client care and outcomes was underscored. Aisha's experience showcased the power of perseverance, compassion, and a steadfast dedication to creating an inclusive, equitable, efficient healthcare system.

Aisha's remarkable journey in cultivating cultural competency at Mercy Mwongozo Hospital and beyond is a powerful testament to the progress made in the healthcare community. Her steadfast dedication to inclusivity and understanding in healthcare settings ignited a deeper, more meaningful conversation about how to serve diverse client populations effectively.

As her endeavours progressed, Aisha shifted towards the upcoming wave of healthcare professionals. She collaborated with local nursing and medical colleges to incorporate cultural competence training into their programs. The early integration of cultural sensitivity in healthcare education played a crucial role in educating future medical professionals to deliver superior clinical care while also being mindful of cultural nuances.

Aisha also initiated a community ambassador program, inviting individuals from diverse ethnic backgrounds to attend regular meetings with healthcare experts. These discussions provided valuable insights into the needs and preferences of different populations, enabling Mercy Mwongozo to tailor its services more effectively. The program also dispelled myths and challenged preconceived notions, fostering a deeper understanding and appreciation among healthcare providers and community members.

Her research centred on the influence of culturally competent care on client outcomes. Through her collaboration with research organisations, Aisha contributed to implementing studies that gathered concrete data on the advantages of cultural competency in healthcare environments. This research contributed to promoting broader policy reforms and increased budget allocation to improve culturally competent practices in healthcare settings.

Aisha's impact also led to the development of client education materials in multiple languages and culturally sensitive health education programs. These materials and programs aimed to provide clients from diverse backgrounds with information and education tailored to their language and cultural needs.

Aisha has facilitated workshops on cultural competency for hospital executives and policymakers. She was convinced that for the healthcare system to achieve effectiveness, it needed to undergo comprehensive changes at every level. Her workshops highlighted the importance of leadership support in establishing an inclusive and culturally sensitive healthcare environment.

Aisha's contributions at Mercy Mwongozo were highly influential. The hospital gained a reputation for its culturally sensitive care, drawing clients from diverse backgrounds seeking a healthcare provider who valued and appreciated their cultural requirements. After training in culturally sensitive care, the hospital staff experienced a heightened sense of fulfilment and confidence in meeting their client's needs.

Aisha's unwavering commitment to promoting cultural competence in healthcare has made her a respected and passionate advocate. She frequently attended international conferences, where she actively engaged in sharing her experiences and perspectives while also gaining valuable insights from fellow experts in the field. She was deeply committed to promoting cultural competence in healthcare, passionately believing that every client should receive care that respects their cultural identity and meets their unique needs.

Mwongozo Hospital and the broader healthcare community underwent a remarkable journey of profound change. It was a tale of triumphing over challenges, fostering empathy, and creating a hospital environment where every client was treated with dignity and compassion. Aisha's ongoing journey and efforts to enhance cultural competence in healthcare serve as a source of inspiration and influence, highlighting the timeless importance of empathy, respect, and inclusivity in the dynamic healthcare industry.

Aisha's commitment to cultural competence profoundly impacted the healthcare landscape, shaping how healthcare providers nationwide approached client care. Her expertise in healthcare garnered the attention of numerous organisations, who sought her guidance on implementing similar programs in their facilities.

She dedicated herself to establishing connections with these organisations, providing them with valuable insights and tools to foster a culture of inclusivity and empathy. Aisha's impact extended well beyond the confines of Mercy Mwongozo Hospital, contributing to a nationwide movement for healthcare that is more attuned to diverse cultural needs.

Aisha got various prizes and distinctions for her work. She found great satisfaction in witnessing tangible improvements in client care and eliminating obstacles to healthcare for diverse communities.

In addition, Aisha's endeavours fostered greater involvement and confidence within the community. Aisha offered a strong voice and support for communities that had previously felt overlooked and misunderstood by the healthcare system. Her efforts to build bridges between these communities and healthcare practitioners resulted in better, more trustworthy relationships, which were critical for effective healthcare delivery.

Her commitment was crucial in reshaping healthcare policies to prioritise diversity and inclusion. Aisha's perspectives, drawn from her extensive field experience, helped policymakers grasp the practical aspects of implementing culturally competent care and its positive influence on client outcomes.

The impact of Aisha's initiatives was also felt in client advocacy. Clients from various backgrounds started to feel more confident in voicing their healthcare needs and preferences, understanding that their opinions would be acknowledged and valued. This advancement was a significant stride in ensuring equitable healthcare for everyone.

Aisha maintained a strong connection with the individuals she assisted while pursuing her profession. She enthusiastically participated in community events and forums, staying informed about different cultural groups' evolving needs and concerns. Her consistent engagement guaranteed that her work remained up-to-date and impactful.

The story of Aisha's tireless dedication to enhancing cultural competence at Mercy Mwongozo Hospital and beyond is a powerful testament to the transformative impact that an individual's unwavering resolve can have on a larger scale. Her journey served as a powerful testament to the effects of healthcare professionals in promoting and implementing procedures that embrace cultural diversity. Aisha's work in cultural competence has been a source of inspiration and guidance, representing a vision of a future where healthcare is inclusive, respectful, and equal for everyone, regardless of their cultural background.

CHAPTER 16

Ethics in the Age of AI

An experienced nurse at Mercy Mwongozo Hospital, Miriam faced a new healthcare challenge: incorporating Artificial Intelligence (AI) into clinical settings. He journeyed into this new realm as the hospital embraced AI-driven diagnostic tools, client monitoring systems, and treatment planning algorithms. Miriam, known for his strong ethical standards and focus on client well-being, approached these changes with curiosity and careful consideration. He immediately grasped the immense advantages that AI could bring to healthcare: enhanced diagnostic precision, tailored treatment approaches, and improved client results. Nevertheless, Miriam was keenly aware of the ethical dilemmas associated with AI. He grappled with complex matters like client privacy, the reliability of AI decisions, and the evolving role of healthcare practitioners in a world that is becoming more computerised.

Miriam dedicatedly educated himself and his coworkers about the application of artificial intelligence in the healthcare industry. He orchestrated workshops and seminars, inviting experts to delve into AI technologies' capabilities, limitations, and ethical considerations. These seminars gave healthcare professionals a valuable opportunity to voice their concerns and gain knowledge about the ethical implementation of AI in client care.

Miriam was deeply committed to ensuring that AI tools were utilised to enhance, rather than supplant, the human element in healthcare. He advocated for a more equitable approach where AI tools improve clinical judgment and decision-making rather than making independent judgments. This approach emphasised the nurse-client interaction and the human intuition that is crucial in healthcare. Miriam also contributed to developing guidelines for the ethical use of artificial intelligence in hospitals. He worked alongside a team of experts in ethics, healthcare, and IT to create protocols that prioritised client consent, data privacy, and transparency when implementing AI-driven solutions. These recommendations set a standard for ethical AI use and serve as a model for other healthcare institutions.

Miriam's curiosity about AI also prompted him to explore its potential for enhancing client education and involvement. He collaborated with technology teams to develop AI-powered instructional tools that gave clients personalised information regarding their ailments and treatments. These technologies helped clients become active participants in their healthcare journey, empowering them to take control of their well-being. His investigation into artificial intelligence in healthcare encompassed client monitoring and follow-up care. He dedicated his efforts to integrating artificial intelligence systems that could analyse client data in real-time, offering early indications of potential health risks. This proactive approach to client care was instrumental in preventing issues and enhancing overall client safety.

Miriam's contributions to navigating the ethical complexities of AI in healthcare are highly influential. He played a crucial role in incorporating AI into the hospital's healthcare system while ensuring its implementation aligned with its core values of client care and ethical conduct. Miriam's journey with AI in healthcare unfolded as a tale of thoughtful adjustment and moral consciousness. It was a story about embracing innovative technologies while staying true to the core principles of healthcare. His journey exemplified how healthcare professionals can pioneer integrating modern technologies into healthcare, ensuring they enhance client care quality and preserve humanity. His expertise in artificial intelligence in healthcare expanded as he played a crucial role in guiding the ethical incorporation of technology in medical practice. His endeavours reached beyond Mercy Mwongozo Hospital, profoundly impacting the overall approach to AI in healthcare.

He started participating in interprofessional forums that gathered healthcare professionals, technologists, ethicists, and client advocates. During these meetings, Miriam highlighted the importance of a multidisciplinary approach to developing and implementing AI technology in healthcare. He was convinced that addressing AI's ethical, practical, and technical challenges necessitated diverse viewpoints. Miriam played a significant role in establishing the standards for client consent in AI applications. He strongly supported the implementation of transparent and comprehensive consent procedures that guaranteed that clients were thoroughly educated about using AI in their healthcare and data collection. These protocols help instil a sense of comfort and security in clients when incorporating AI into their healthcare journey.

Miriam understood the significance of consistently monitoring and evaluating AI systems. It is essential to regularly assess AI applications in clinical contexts to evaluate their impact on client care, accuracy, and efficacy. These audits ensured AI technologies met the most rigorous healthcare delivery and ethical practice standards. He stayed deeply engaged in client care, utilising AI techniques with a considerate and client-focused approach alongside his efforts in policy and implementation. He used AI-driven data to enhance his clinical decision-making, consistently prioritising human judgment in the final decision on client care while being informed by AI analysis.

Miriam's journey in artificial intelligence and healthcare has inspired him to guide and support aspiring healthcare professionals. He educated them on the potential and advantages of artificial intelligence in healthcare while emphasising the ethical responsibilities accompanying these powerful tools. He fostered a sense of duty in them to utilise technology with care and empathy, prioritising the well-being and dignity of clients above all else.

Miriam's work with artificial intelligence in healthcare at Mercy Mwongozo Hospital served as a compelling demonstration of the harmonious coexistence of technology and ethics in the medical industry. It highlighted the significance of healthcare professionals as mediators and mentors in the ethical implementation of technology. His journey was a touching tale of how understanding, moral thought, and technological progress can collaborate to create a more sophisticated and empathetic future of healthcare. Miriam's thoughtful approach to artificial intelligence in healthcare has consistently served as a source of inspiration and guidance, setting a benchmark for healthcare professionals to effectively navigate the complex intersection of technology, ethics, and client care. Miriam's deep engagement with AI in healthcare transformed Mercy Hospital's operations and sparked discussions within the broader medical community. He gained recognition for his fair and moral approach to implementing AI technology, ensuring that it improved client care quality instead of diminishing it.

Through his commitment to the responsible use of AI, he fostered collaboration with technology developers. Miriam provided valuable perspectives on the practical needs of healthcare professionals and clients, guaranteeing that new AI solutions were developed with a focus on clients' well-being. His involvement in these collaborations ensured that AI tools were not only cutting-edge in technology but also considered ethical considerations and addressed the needs of healthcare providers and clients. Miriam's research highlighted the significance of transparency in AI algorithms utilised in healthcare settings. He advocated for developing AI systems that healthcare providers could understand and trust. Transparency plays a crucial role in building trust in AI tools among healthcare professionals and clients, establishing these tools as reliable assistants in healthcare provision.

Miriam also initiated a series of community outreach programs to enlighten the public about the application of AI in healthcare. He made a case for the importance of informing clients about the potential applications of artificial intelligence (AI) in their healthcare. These programs assisted clients in gaining a better understanding of AI by addressing common concerns and questions while offering valuable insights into how AI is improving healthcare.

Miriam's influence reached far and wide, shaping the development of national policies. He actively participated in panels and committees that set guidelines for artificial intelligence in healthcare, advocating for regulations prioritising client safety and privacy. His contributions were instrumental in shaping national policies regarding the use of AI in healthcare, with a strong emphasis on ethical considerations. Miriam utilised AI tools to tailor client care in his ongoing work at Mercy Mwongozo. He was involved in cutting-edge technologies that processed vast client data to provide tailored therapy recommendations. The AI-powered recommendations combined Miriam's clinical experience to ensure that each client received personalised care based on their unique needs.

Miriam also recognised the immense potential of AI in predicting healthcare outcomes. He was involved in projects utilising artificial intelligence to analyse patterns in client data, predict potential health issues, and facilitate proactive healthcare. This predictive technique had significant implications for preventive medicine, enabling healthcare practitioners to intervene earlier and more efficiently manage health concerns. Miriam's work in AI in healthcare significantly impacted various aspects. He played a crucial part in incorporating AI into the hospital's healthcare system and was instrumental in setting ethical guidelines for its implementation. His thoughtful approach to artificial intelligence in healthcare served as a model for other institutions, showcasing how technology can enhance client care while upholding ethical standards.

Miriam's experience with AI in healthcare at Mercy Mwongozo Hospital exemplifies a remarkable tale of forward-thinking and conscientious technology integration in medicine. It was a narrative that delved into navigating the obstacles and possibilities presented by artificial intelligence while upholding a steadfast dedication to client well-being and ethical conduct. His contributions have been a source of inspiration and guidance, playing a crucial role in shaping the future of healthcare at a time when the intersection of technology and ethics is more prominent than ever. Miriam's approach to artificial intelligence in healthcare sets a standard for how healthcare practitioners can embrace technological advancements while prioritising client care and medical ethics.

Miriam's endeavours at Mercy Mwongozo Hospital to incorporate AI into healthcare started to make waves in the broader healthcare industry. He rapidly gained recognition as a highly sought-after speaker and consultant, sharing his knowledge and insights on AI in healthcare at numerous forums and organisations. Miriam highlighted the importance of adopting a well-rounded approach to AI in these interactions, combining technology's accuracy with the invaluable human element in healthcare.

Through his dedication to promoting the responsible application of AI, he successfully established a certification program specifically designed for AI technologies in the healthcare industry. This program evaluates AI applications using various criteria, including accuracy, transparency, ethical considerations, and alignment with client care objectives. Miriam's involvement in this program contributed to developing industry-wide standards for AI tools, guaranteeing their adherence to the highest quality and ethical benchmarks.

Miriam focused on cultivating a healthcare workforce well-versed in AI and endeavours in AI technologies. He thought it was important for all healthcare professionals to understand artificial intelligence, including its potential uses and ethical considerations. With this aim in mind, he developed training modules and tools that ensured AI education was accessible to every employee at Mercy Mwongozo Hospital. These educational activities gave healthcare practitioners the necessary knowledge to make well-informed decisions regarding using AI. Miriam delved into AI to explore its potential to enhance the client experience and foster greater engagement. He collaborated with technology teams to develop AI-powered client portals that provided personalised health information and interactive health and wellness management tools. These portals serve as a valuable resource for clients, empowering them to actively engage in their healthcare journey.

Miriam's research delved into the ethical considerations surrounding client data management in artificial intelligence. He strongly advocated stringent data privacy measures, prioritising client data protection and secure management in AI applications. His contributions in this field have significantly increased awareness about the importance of data security in the era of digital healthcare. Miriam's efforts had a significant influence across the entire hospital.

Staff members developed a greater sense of assurance in utilising AI technologies, resulting in enhanced client care that is tailored and more efficient. As a result, the hospital's healthcare delivery system experienced notable improvements.

Miriam's dedication persisted as he remained a passionate advocate for the responsible application of AI in healthcare. He remained well-informed about the latest AI advancements, consistently exploring their potential to enhance client care with an unwavering commitment to ethical principles. His work with AI in healthcare at Mercy Mwongozo Hospital is a remarkable testament to the power of ethical innovation. It highlighted the crucial role that healthcare professionals play in shaping the incorporation of technology in medicine. Miriam's journey was a powerful reminder of the importance of balancing technical advancement and fundamental healthcare principles. It emphasised the significance of always keeping sight of the values of compassion, ethics, and client-centred care in the pursuit of progress.

CHAPTER 17

The Policy Arena

Now in a leadership position at Mercy Mwongozo Hospital, Zara faced a new challenge beyond the hospital's boundaries. She embarked on her first significant foray into policy advocacy when she was assigned to address a pressing healthcare issue that had implications for her town and the entire state. The issue was a severe lack of nursing staff, significantly impacting regional client care.

Zara was compelled to take action due to her extensive experience in nursing and newfound position of influence. She assembled a coalition of healthcare experts from different hospitals and healthcare organisations, which included nurses, doctors, and administrators. This collaboration sought to increase awareness about the nursing shortage and advocate for measures to address this critical issue.

Zara spearheaded an initiative to gather evidence and data to support the coalition's argument. They conducted surveys, collected client care and outcomes statistics, and interviewed healthcare workers and clients. This information provided a grim outlook on the effects of the nursing shortage, including extended hospital stays, increased client readmissions, and a decline in the quality of client care.

Equipped with this knowledge, Zara and her alliance approached state legislators, presenting a compelling case for legislative changes to address the nursing shortage. They advocated for more significant funding for nursing education programs, financial incentives to attract and retain nursing professionals, and regulatory reforms to enable nurses to practice to their fullest potential.

Zara understood the significance of gaining support from the masses. She orchestrated public forums and media campaigns to raise awareness of the issue. The coalition's efforts garnered significant media attention, leading to widespread public and political debate surrounding the nursing shortage.

Zara encountered numerous challenges during this process, including political challenges, internal disagreements within the alliance, and the intricate nature of transforming a complex system like healthcare. However, her strong leadership, determination, and unwavering commitment to the cause ensured that the momentum continued.

During the campaign, Zara held several vital meetings with legislators, demonstrating her ability to be a strong advocate for healthcare issues. She recounted stories of clients and healthcare professionals affected by the nursing shortage rather than simply presenting statistics and numbers.

The lobbying efforts started to show results. Legislative bills were introduced to address some of the coalition's suggestions. Zara and her team put in a great effort, offering their insights and opinions on proposed legislation and persistently advocating for the measures until they were successfully passed.

Zara's initial policy lobbying concern showcased her strong leadership and unwavering commitment to enhancing healthcare. It was a journey that took her from Mercy Mwongozo to the hallways of the state capitol, showcasing the significant impact healthcare workers can have on legislation.

Zara's advocacy story has emerged as a captivating illustration of how healthcare professionals can expand their impact beyond client care and into policy and legislation. Her journey exemplified nurses' and healthcare professionals' crucial role in shaping healthcare policy and ensuring the healthcare system meets the needs of all stakeholders with compassion and effectiveness.

Zara's career in policy gained momentum as she solidified her position as a respected figure in healthcare advocacy. She achieved significant legislative improvements through her dedication to addressing the nursing shortage issue and gained recognition as a prominent advocate for healthcare professionals. As her popularity grew, Zara expanded her focus on other essential healthcare issues, broadening the range of her advocacy efforts.

Her next focus was to enhance client access to healthcare. Zara spearheaded initiatives to identify and eliminate obstacles to ensure the community has proper access to healthcare. She actively engaged with community leaders, healthcare providers, and clients to better understand their finances, geography, and cultural concerns.

Zara and her colleagues formulated policy recommendations to enhance healthcare accessibility following a comprehensive analysis of these constraints. These suggestions encompassed the need for additional funding in healthcare for disadvantaged regions, the expansion of insurance coverage, and the implementation of community-based health initiatives. She engaged in discussions with lawmakers, presenting thoroughly researched ideas and garnering support from the medical community and the Mwongozo public.

Zara's activism in this area showcased her knack for engaging with individuals from diverse backgrounds and industries. She fostered collaboration among various stakeholders, cultivating relationships crucial in advocating for impactful policy reforms. Her ability to promote agreement and inspire teamwork was essential to the achievements of her endeavours.

Zara also acknowledged the importance of innovation in healthcare. She advocated for policies that supported the progress of healthcare technologies and therapies. She aspired to create an accessible healthcare system at the forefront of innovation, providing clients with the highest-quality care.

Zara's efforts started to make a noticeable difference in shaping policy reforms. The number of healthcare professionals entering the field significantly rose, resulting in enhanced client access to healthcare services and improved quality of care. These reforms showcased significant advancements in addressing the healthcare industry's most urgent issues.

Zara was strongly dedicated to her nursing background as she pursued her professional journey. She ensured that nurses' perspectives and insights were included in policy discussions. Her influential lobbying and vigorous leadership activities catalysed other healthcare professionals, motivating them to actively engage in policy and advocacy efforts to enhance the healthcare system.

Zara's work in policy at Mercy Mwongozo Hospital and elsewhere is a testament to her strong leadership and unwavering commitment to advancing healthcare. The example showcased the influence of lobbying in bringing about change and the crucial involvement of healthcare professionals in shaping policies that promote community health and well-being. Zara's experience in policy advocacy has been truly inspiring, highlighting the significance of actively engaging in policymaking to create a healthcare system that is both fair and efficient.

Zara's policy role developed as she tackled increasingly complex and far-reaching healthcare issues. It became evident that she deeply understood the intricate maze of healthcare policy and was committed to enacting substantial changes. She began dedicating her efforts to national initiatives, with a focus on significant healthcare improvements that have the potential to benefit people across the entire country.

One of her notable achievements was advocating for reforms in mental health care. Zara observed the increasing need for enhanced mental health treatments and disparities in their availability. She took the lead in an initiative to incorporate mental health treatment into primary care settings, expanding the reach of mental health services to a broader community.

Her efforts in this field encompassed advocating for increased funding for mental health services and the destigmatisation of mental health. Zara hosted conferences and public speaking events where she delved into the significance of mental health, presenting personal stories and compelling evidence highlighting the urgency for comprehensive reform in mental healthcare.

Zara is dedicated to enhancing client safety standards in healthcare institutions, alongside her efforts in mental health. She collaborated with healthcare professionals, client safety experts, and lawmakers to develop new safety rules and recommendations. Through her diligent work, she successfully implemented stricter safety protocols, decreasing medical mistakes and improving the overall quality of client care.

Zara also acknowledged the importance of technology in revolutionising healthcare. She advocated for implementing legislation that promotes the adoption of digital health technologies, such as electronic health records and telemedicine services. Her objective was to enhance healthcare efficiency and accessibility, especially for individuals residing in remote or disadvantaged regions.

Her expertise and influence allowed her to participate in various global health initiatives. Zara collaborated with international organisations to improve healthcare systems in underprivileged nations. She utilised her knowledge and understanding to contribute to these projects, aiding in creating sustainable and culturally sensitive healthcare solutions.

Zara maintained regular communication with her colleagues from Mercy Mwongozo Hospital throughout her career in policy advocacy. She often came back to discuss her perspectives and experiences, motivating others to delve into the influence they could have outside of direct client care. Her stories and achievements served as a source of inspiration for numerous employees at Mercy Mwongozo, motivating them to engage actively in healthcare advocacy and policy.

Zara's lobbying efforts faced numerous challenges. She often faced resistance and bureaucratic obstacles. Her determination and skill in building relationships and finding common understanding allowed her to conquer these obstacles. She gained recognition for her diplomatic skills and knack for navigating intricate political landscapes to accomplish her goals.

Zara's work in policy had significant and wide-ranging implications. Her valuable contributions significantly improved the lives of numerous individuals as she worked towards making healthcare more accessible, safe, and compassionate. Her actions also laid the foundation for future healthcare changes, showcasing the impact that dedicated and driven healthcare workers can have on policy.

Zara's story of policy advocacy at Mercy Mwongozo Hospital and beyond was an impressive demonstration of her strong leadership skills and unwavering commitment to improving public health. Her journey showcased healthcare professionals' ability to impact the healthcare system significantly. Zara's story has been a source of inspiration and motivation, emphasising the critical role of healthcare professionals in advocating for healthcare legislation and striving for a healthcare system that is inclusive and compassionate towards all individuals.

Zara's policy advocacy profoundly impacted the upcoming generation of healthcare professionals. Appreciating the importance of policy comprehension in healthcare, she implemented initiatives at Mercy Mwongozo Hospital to educate nurses and doctors about health policy and advocacy. Engaging in seminars, workshops, and guest lectures with policymakers and healthcare activists was integral to these programs. She aimed to cultivate a strong sense of accountability and capability in healthcare professionals, empowering them to shape and engage in policy-making processes that impact their field.

Zara's engagement in policy advocacy activities also led her to establish partnerships with academic institutions. She contributed to developing health policy courses by integrating practical issues and solutions into the curriculum. This integration helped bridge the divide between theoretical knowledge and real-world policy implementation, equipping students with the skills to become effective advocates in their future careers.

Zara's extensive experience in policy lobbying has influenced her perspective on healthcare, leading her to develop a more holistic and all-encompassing approach. She understood the importance of implementing policies that consider physical health and social and environmental factors impacting overall well-being. Her activism expanded to encompass the social determinants of health, including housing, nutrition, and education, all of which play a crucial role in achieving complete health equity.

Zara's work also involved championing diversity and inclusion in healthcare legislation. She strongly supported policies to provide universal healthcare access, regardless of one's financial background. She placed great importance on promoting inclusivity, not only by granting access but also by ensuring that healthcare services were attuned to the diverse needs of individuals.

Zara's work had a significant impact due to the positive improvements she contributed to. Her knack for transforming intricate healthcare issues into practical policy enhancements showcased her exceptional aptitude and determination. Her advocacy significantly impacted policies that enhanced healthcare delivery, access, and quality, benefiting clients and providers.

Zara consistently advocated for healthcare practices, prioritising clients' needs throughout her professional journey. She believed that all policy decisions should prioritise the well-being of clients. Her unwavering commitment to this principle permeated her work. It ignited a sense of introspection among those in her healthcare profession, encouraging them to ponder the broader ramifications of their roles.

Zara's work at Mercy Mwongozo Hospital and in the broader healthcare community was marked by visionary leadership and unwavering dedication to enhancing public health. Her journey was a powerful reminder of healthcare professionals' significant impact in shaping the regulations that govern their work and the lives of countless individuals. Zara's advocacy efforts have consistently been a source of inspiration and guidance, emphasising the crucial importance of engaging in healthcare policy to ensure a healthcare system that is fair, efficient, and compassionate.

CHAPTER 18

Mental Health Frontlines

John, an experienced nurse at Mercy Mwongozo Hospital, identified a previously overlooked healthcare concern: nurses' mental well-being. Having personally observed the immense pressure and emotional strain that nursing can impose, John decided to initiate a specialised mental health program for nurses.

He initiated a series of open forums and conversations at the hospital, providing a safe space for nurses to express their experiences, issues, and concerns. These conversations highlighted the importance of offering better support and resources for the mental well-being of healthcare professionals.

John created a thorough mental health program, drawing from the knowledge gained in these sessions. He aimed to develop a comprehensive support system encompassing counselling, stress management training, and peer support groups. He collaborated with mental health professionals to tailor the program to address nurses' specific challenges.

John actively advocated for policy changes at the institution. He tirelessly dedicated himself to enlightening hospital administrators about the importance of nursing mental health. Through his efforts, he successfully advocated for implementing policies that strongly emphasised mental health, including the introduction of routine mental health check-ins and dedicated mental health days.

John's mental health program also offers workshops on identifying signs of burnout and strategies for managing it. These courses were designed to equip nurses with the necessary knowledge and resources to prioritise their mental well-being actively.

Furthermore, John implemented a mentorship program as a component of the mental health initiative. Experienced nurses were paired with new employees to offer guidance, assistance, and a compassionate ear. This mentorship program helped foster a culture of empathy and understanding among the nursing staff, enhancing the sense of community and support.

John's campaign highlighted the importance of addressing workplace mental health issues without judgment. He demonstrated a commendable approach by openly sharing his experiences and encouraging others to do the same. This openness fostered a transformation in the mental health discourse within the hospital, leading to its increased acceptance and open discussion.

John's program for nurses' mental health had a profound effect. Nurses at Mercy Mwongozo Hospital expressed a sense of increased support and decreased anxiety. Job satisfaction rose significantly, and burnout rates decreased significantly. The program positively impacted both the nurses and the quality of client care. Nurses became better prepared, both emotionally and mentally, to handle the challenges of their profession.

John's work at Mercy Mwongozo Hospital in developing the mental health program for nurses is a remarkable tale of compassion, resilience, and practical guidance. The importance of mental health support in the healthcare profession and its positive impact on healthcare personnel and clients was highlighted. John's experience showcased the power of individual drive in bringing about significant enhancements in the workplace, fostering a more nurturing and conducive environment for everyone involved.

John's mental health program for nurses has gained significant recognition beyond Mercy Mwongozo Hospital, becoming a widely respected model for other healthcare facilities. He was invited to speak at multiple healthcare conferences and seminars to share his experiences and discuss the program's success. His discussions offered valuable perspectives on the implementation and benefits of such initiatives, inspiring other medical facilities to adopt similar approaches.

The program's success at Mercy Mwongozo resulted in collaboration with nursing schools and healthcare organisations. John worked closely with these organisations to incorporate mental health awareness and self-care practices into nursing education and training programs. He was convinced that equipping young nurses with these tools right from the beginning of their careers was crucial for fostering long-term well-being and resilience.

John emphasised the importance of implementing a culture transformation within the hospital in addition to the planned components of the program. He created a culture that encouraged and supported employees in seeking mental health care, fostering an environment where they felt comfortable discussing their mental well-being without any fear of being stigmatised or judged. This cultural shift played a crucial role in altering perspectives on mental health within the medical community.

John also understood the importance of consistently evaluating and improving the mental health program. He created a feedback system that allows nurses to share their experiences and suggest improvements to the program. This continuous feedback loop ensured that the program stayed up-to-date, efficient, and adaptable to nurses' evolving needs.

The mental health program also included annual retreats and workshops on self-care, mindfulness, and relaxation techniques. These gatherings allowed nurses to unwind, reflect, and recharge, benefiting their overall well-being.

Mercy Mwongozo Hospital's mental health program flourished under John's exceptional leadership as a source of support and empathy for nurses. It not only fulfilled the immediate needs of the nursing staff but also sparked a broader conversation about the importance of mental health in the healthcare sector.

John's experience creating and overseeing a mental health program for nurses was marked by compassion, creativity, and dedication. It highlighted the crucial role that healthcare leaders can play in tackling workplace mental health. John's unwavering commitment to his colleagues' mental well-being inspires and influences him. It reinforces the importance of providing comprehensive care for healthcare workers, ensuring they receive the necessary physical and psychological support to fulfil their vital responsibilities.

John's efforts at Mercy Mwongozo Hospital set a new standard, and his commitment to the well-being of nurses had a significant impact on the healthcare industry. The success of the mental health program ignited a broader movement to champion the mental well-being of healthcare professionals from various fields.

Appreciating the program's significant influence, John expanded its scope to encompass additional healthcare personnel within the hospital. He acknowledged the shared challenges and barriers experienced by nurses, physicians, technicians, and support personnel. This inclusive strategy, which offered comprehensive mental health care to all hospital staff, broadened the program's scope.

The extended program included several sessions focused on building resilience. These programs were designed to educate healthcare professionals on effective stress management, resilience, and healthy work-life balance. The interactive nature of these seminars encouraged active engagement and the exchange of personal insights, enhancing the staff's sense of camaraderie and assistance.

Furthermore, John advocated incorporating mental health awareness into the hospital's safety and wellness policies. He collaborated with the hospital's human resources department to prioritise mental health in the workplace, placing it on par with physical health. As a result of this integration, policies were developed to support frequent mental health check-ups, confidential counselling services, and proactive interventions.

In addition, John's program started to prioritise early intervention. He implemented regular assessments to gauge burnout and stress levels among hospital staff. He recognised these signs early on and allowed for prompt assistance and intervention, averting more severe mental health challenges.

The program's achievements at Mercy Mwongozo prompted collaboration with healthcare officials. John was invited to participate in national healthcare policy talks, where he passionately advocated for the inclusion of mental health support for healthcare personnel. His keen insights contributed to formulating policies that acknowledged and tackled the mental health requirements of healthcare professionals.

John's efforts also garnered the interest of scholars. He collaborated with scholars to study the effects of the mental health program on employee performance, client care, and overall hospital efficiency. The research findings provided concrete evidence of the advantages of prioritising the mental well-being of healthcare professionals, thus supporting the importance of implementing such programs.

Under John's guidance, the mental health program became a benchmark for other hospitals and healthcare facilities. It went

167

beyond its initial purpose and became a movement, shedding light on a frequently neglected aspect of healthcare professionals' well-being. John's approach, characterised by understanding, proactive assistance, and ongoing enhancement, set a new benchmark in mental health support within the healthcare industry.

John's experience with Mercy Mwongozo Hospital's mental health program was characterised by empathy and firm guidance. The text highlighted the importance of acknowledging and addressing the mental health requirements of individuals who dedicate themselves to the well-being of others. His dedication and passion for this cause remain a driving force, highlighting the importance of prioritising the mental well-being of healthcare professionals to better the healthcare system as a whole. John's endeavours exemplified the notion that a healthcare system that prioritises the well-being of its practitioners is more adept at providing quality care to its clients. As a result, his journey has impacted the realm of healthcare.

John's efforts to promote mental health awareness have grown, becoming a significant part of the hospital's culture. He advocated integrating mental health training and practice into all healthcare education and practice aspects. This holistic approach ensured that new healthcare professionals joining Mercy Mwongozo were immediately immersed in an environment that values mental well-being.

Aside from participating in internal programs, John also dedicated his time to volunteering in the community. He created outreach programs to combat the negative perception of mental health in healthcare. Public seminars, community workshops, and collaborations with local media were used to communicate stories and knowledge regarding the significance of mental health for healthcare personnel.

His commitment to this cause led to a digital platform - a hub where healthcare professionals could access mental health information, share experiences, and seek assistance. This website provides a safe and inclusive space for healthcare professionals from different locations to connect and offer mutual support.

John's lobbying efforts led to a deeper understanding of the mental health challenges faced by healthcare practitioners. He played a crucial role in fostering a culture that promoted open discussions about mental health and encouraged seeking treatment as a sign of strength rather than weakness.

John's efforts led to an increase in morale and a decrease in burnout rates among the personnel at Mercy Mwongozo. Healthcare professionals expressed greater appreciation and encouragement, enhancing client care and a more positive work environment.

In addition, John's ideas started to influence policy significantly on a broader scale. Healthcare providers and governments began acknowledging the essential requirement for mental health services in healthcare settings. John's contribution was crucial in this transformation, as other hospitals and healthcare organisations adopted his model for mental health support.

John was dedicated to promoting mental health and constantly sought new approaches to enhance the well-being of healthcare professionals. His story became a testament to the profound impact of understanding, guidance, and unwavering support.

John's story at Mercy Mwongozo Hospital showcased the remarkable impact that an individual's vision and unwavering commitment can have on advancing mental health awareness and support within the healthcare industry. It is a powerful reminder of the potential for significant progress in our healthcare system. His experience was a powerful reminder of the importance of supporting those dedicated to creating a more compassionate and efficient healthcare environment for everyone.

CHAPTER 19

Grace's Tender Care

Grace, a nurse at Mercy Mwongozo Hospital, embarked on a mission to revolutionise how elderly individuals receive care. She embarked on a journey driven by a profound understanding: elderly individuals need more than just medical treatment; they deserve emotional assistance, preservation of their dignity, and recognition of their life journeys.

Grace started by developing a thorough care program tailored to the unique needs of elderly clients, driven by a strong passion for having a positive impact. This program took a holistic approach, addressing not just the physical health of older people but also their mental and emotional well-being.

Including individualised care plans was a crucial element of Grace's program. She dedicated herself to understanding clients' backgrounds, preferences, and life experiences. The data was utilised to create care plans that were medically accurate and held personal significance. This approach facilitated a deeper connection between individuals receiving care and their careers.

Grace also presented a variety of therapeutic exercises designed to enhance the cognitive and emotional well-being of older individuals. Engaging in music therapy, art classes, and memory exercises proved enjoyable and effective in slowing the clients' cognitive function decline.

Grace prioritised creating a nurturing and stimulating atmosphere within the hospital's senior care unit. She transformed the space with vibrant colours, cosy furniture, and abundant natural light. The complex also featured gardens and walking routes, allowing clients to enjoy the outdoors in a secure and appealing environment.

Grace's approach was also innovative in its focus on involving the entire family. She encouraged family members to actively engage in the care process by providing information and support to help them comprehend and contribute to caring for their elderly loved ones.

Grace also understood the importance of training staff members working with elderly clients. She facilitated workshops and training sessions focused on the needs of older people, including effective communication strategies, recognising common age-related conditions, and addressing the emotional challenges of ageing.

She actively collaborated with other hospital departments. Grace worked alongside dietitians, physiotherapists, and mental health professionals to ensure a comprehensive and multidisciplinary approach to aged care. This collaboration ensured that every aspect of an elderly client's well-being was considered.

Grace's program had a profound impact. Clients in the senior care unit experienced significant improvements in their physical and emotional well-being. They shared a sense of appreciation, compassion, and empathy. The personnel experienced greater fulfilment in their employment, thanks to their knowledge and skills in delivering high-quality, compassionate care.

Grace's unique approach to caring for elderly clients at Mercy Mwongozo Hospital was a heartwarming tale of compassion, creativity, and comprehensive care. It showcased the impact of thoughtful, person-focused care on older individuals. Her experience showcased the ability of healthcare professionals to go above and beyond standard medical care, enhancing the well-being of elderly clients and ensuring their final years are filled with dignity, happiness, and reverence.

Grace's innovative approach to caring for older clients quickly gained recognition throughout Mercy Mwongozo Hospital, establishing a fresh benchmark for geriatric care. Her program not only enhanced the well-being of elderly clients, but it also served as a blueprint for other hospital departments, fostering a more holistic and empathetic approach to client care for individuals of all generations.

Grace was sought after to present her ideas at various healthcare forums and conferences due to her program's remarkable success and impact. Her speeches, with practical advice and inspiring success stories, motivated other healthcare professionals to adopt similar approaches in their organisations. Grace's work was starting to make waves in the broader field of geriatric care as she pushed for reforms in treating elderly clients across the healthcare system.

Grace diligently worked on her program at Mercy Mwongozo while juggling her other commitments. She initiated a volunteer program, inviting community members to dedicate their time to elderly clients. These dedicated individuals, ranging from students to seniors, offered companionship and interaction to the clients, further enhancing their daily experiences.

Grace was also intrigued by the potential of technology to enhance senior care. She introduced telemedicine services to cater to clients who couldn't attend the hospital for regular check-ups. This not only made healthcare more accessible but also facilitated continuous monitoring and support for elderly individuals in their homes.

Grace's commitment to caring for older people extended to providing support during their final stages of life. She worked closely with the palliative care team to ensure that elderly individuals received compassionate and dignified treatment during their last days. Her approach focused on providing effective pain management, offering emotional support, and respecting the client's desires and independence.

The program's impact was evident in the feedback received from the clients' families. They expressed their appreciation for the thoughtful and attentive care provided to their loved ones, emphasising the positive improvements in their overall health. Family members were highly engaged and well-informed, which cultivated a strong sense of collaboration and confidence with the healthcare staff.

Grace was strongly dedicated to continuous learning and personal development as she advanced her career. She stayed up to date on geriatric care research, constantly seeking innovative methods to enhance the well-being of older individuals. Her unwavering dedication to aged care stemmed from her deep conviction in the inherent value and respect owed to every individual, regardless of age.

Grace's narrative about her experience in elderly client care at Mercy Mwongozo Hospital served as a powerful testament to the profound influence that empathetic and inventive care can have on the lives of older individuals. Her story showcased the deep influence healthcare professionals can have on clients' lives, ensuring their later years are filled with dignity, comfort, and happiness. Grace's innovative approach to senior care has consistently sparked inspiration and provided guidance, setting a fresh benchmark in aged care and highlighting the vital contribution of healthcare professionals in enhancing the well-being of older individuals.

Grace's innovative work in elderly client care at Mercy Mwongozo Hospital swiftly captured the interest of healthcare policymakers and geriatric medicine specialists. Her approach, seamlessly blending empathetic care with cutting-edge advancements in medicine and technology, was celebrated as a prime example of geriatric innovation.

Due to her notable achievements, Grace was invited to join national panels focused on enhancing aged care nationwide. She strongly supported legislation prioritising older people's overall health and happiness in these settings. Her impact was instrumental in creating national initiatives to deliver comprehensive and respectful care to older people.

Grace returned to Mercy Mwongozo and continued to enhance her program. She created memory care facilities specifically tailored to individuals with dementia and Alzheimer's disease. These units were staffed by highly knowledgeable healthcare professionals, who made a therapeutic atmosphere that was secure, compassionate, and mentally engaging for individuals with cognitive impairments.

Grace also supported the implementation of non-pharmacological methods in senior care. She integrated pet therapy, gardening, and storytelling into the clients' daily routines. These activities not only brought joy and excitement to clients but also contributed to a decrease in the reliance on medication for managing behavioural and psychological symptoms of dementia.

Grace's program's success resulted in Mercy Mwongozo's recognition as a centre of excellence in senior care. The hospital was transformed into a training facility for specialists in geriatric medicine. Medical professionals from all over the country eagerly came to Mercy Mwongozo to learn from Grace's program, aspiring to replicate its achievements in their environments.

Grace also emphasised the importance of family support and education. She regularly hosted seminars for family members of older clients, offering them guidance and valuable resources on supporting their ageing loved ones. These meetings provided families with the necessary information and support to make well-informed decisions about the care of their loved ones.

Grace always focused on addressing every client's unique requirement as she strived to improve senior care. She dedicated herself to spending quality time with each of her clients, attentively listening to their stories and gaining insight into their unique preferences. This individualised approach ensured that every client felt valued and esteemed, enhancing their overall health.

Grace's journey at Mercy Mwongozo Hospital in transforming old client care was marked by empathy, creativity, and steadfast support for the elderly. Her work extended beyond conventional medical treatment, highlighting the importance of holistic and individualised care for older people. Her program not only enhanced the well-being of elderly individuals, but it also set new benchmarks in geriatric care, motivating healthcare professionals to view senior care as a specialised field that requires innovation, compassion, and a comprehensive understanding of the ageing process.

Grace's innovative approach to aged care has consistently sparked inspiration and left a lasting impact, shaping a future where older people are valued and cared for with utmost dignity, respect, and empathy. Her work highlighted the importance of recognising older people's unique experiences and needs, emphasising the significance of providing care that enhances their well-being and acknowledges their valuable contributions to society.

Grace's unique perspective on senior care started to profoundly affect not just Mercy Mwongozo Hospital's operations but also the larger conversation surrounding ageing and healthcare. She emerged as a passionate advocate for reframing the conversation around ageing, highlighting older individuals' untapped potential and vitality instead of viewing ageing as a mere decline.

Through her dedication, she successfully established community outreach programs that fostered social and educational engagement among older people. These programs aimed to promote a sense of community and purpose among older people, encouraging their integration into society. Grace was pivotal in fostering a more inclusive environment that allowed the elderly to flourish by bridging the gap between the hospital and the community.

Grace played a crucial role in initiating research studies to explore the lasting effects of her comprehensive care approach. She contributed to gathering data on client outcomes, quality of life, and the program's overall success through partnerships with universities and research institutions. The research findings offered valuable insights into best practices in aged care and highlighted the importance of Grace's approach.

Grace incorporated input from clients, relatives, and staff to further enhance the program's ongoing development, driven by her unwavering pursuit of improvement. This feedback loop ensured that the care provided was focused on the client's needs, responsive, and aligned with the latest advancements in geriatric care.

Grace recognised the importance of addressing the spiritual needs of elderly clients. She worked alongside local spiritual leaders and counsellors to provide spiritual guidance and support to clients who sought it. Clients and their families found this aspect of treatment to be especially valuable as it catered to the comprehensive needs of older people.

Grace's program's success led to partnerships with other healthcare centres and nursing homes. These collaborations fostered the sharing of valuable insights and resources, amplifying the influence of Grace's efforts.

Grace stayed grounded and dedicated to providing outstanding care to older people as her reputation grew. She continued actively involved in her role, regularly engaging with clients and their families and guiding her team.

Grace's work in aged care at Mercy Mwongozo Hospital is a testament to her remarkable dedication and expertise in geriatric care. Her journey was a powerful reminder to recognise older people as individuals with distinct needs and diverse experiences rather than as a homogeneous collective. Grace's innovative approach to elderly care has consistently sparked inspiration and provided guidance, shaping the perception and delivery of elderly care. It highlights the profound effect that compassionate and comprehensive care can have on the lives of older individuals.

CHAPTER 20

The Burnout Epidemic

Noah, a diligent nurse at Mercy Mwongozo Hospital, noticed a growing concern among his colleagues - the problem of burnout. Recognising the demanding nature of the healthcare profession and the potential emotional strain it can cause, Noah felt a pressing need to confront this issue directly. He aimed to initiate a dialogue within the hospital regarding professional stress and burnout to shed light on this often-delicate topic.

He initiated a series of informal staff gatherings, providing a safe space for individuals to share their work experiences and emotions openly. These gatherings quickly gained popularity as they allowed healthcare workers to openly discuss their concerns without fear of criticism or reprisal. Noah worked with hospital administration to thoroughly evaluate job stress and burnout, acknowledging the importance of a more structured approach. The findings were surprising, revealing notable employee stress and fatigue levels. With this knowledge, Noah advocated for structural reforms to tackle these obstacles.

He proposed the establishment of a wellness committee to tackle the mental and physical well-being of the hospital staff. This committee, comprised of officials from various departments, was responsible for developing strategies and initiatives to address burnout and foster a more conducive work environment. Noah initiated one of the committee's initial endeavours, organising regular wellness workshops. These sessions focused on techniques for managing stress, practising mindfulness, and prioritising self-care. They were designed to cater to the needs of all hospital staff, acknowledging the widespread impact of burnout in the healthcare sector.

Noah emphasised the importance of effective leadership when managing stress in the workplace. He conducted training workshops for hospital executives and managers, educating them on identifying signs of burnout in their teams and fostering a supportive and transparent work environment. This training helped foster a sense of empathy and comprehension among the hospital's leadership.

Noah advocated for changes in scheduling and personnel regulations. He acknowledged that extended work hours and inadequate staffing contributed to burnout. He was crucial in implementing a more flexible scheduling system, advocating for hiring additional workers to alleviate the strain, and collaborating closely with hospital management. Noah's hard work started to pay off. Employees expressed a sense of increased support and reduced anxiety. The work environment experienced a significant improvement as employees began to engage in more collaborative efforts and enhance their communication skills.

Noah's effort to start a discussion about workplace stress at Mercy Mwongozo Hospital developed into a narrative of understanding, change, and assistance. His narrative emphasised the significance of taking proactive measures to tackle burnout in the healthcare sector. His dedication to raising awareness and implementing practical solutions continued to inspire and foster a culture of well-being and support within the hospital, highlighting the critical role of healthcare professionals in shaping client care and their colleagues' overall well-being. Noah's project at Mercy Mwongozo Hospital had a profound effect that extended far beyond the initial discussions and workshops. His efforts ignited a broader movement within the hospital, advocating for a more comprehensive approach to staff well-being and job satisfaction.

Appreciating the intricacies of burnout, Noah collaborated with mental health professionals to establish a support system within a hospital setting. This system offered confidential counselling services for employees needing expert support for stress and mental health challenges. Noah significantly promoted the acceptance of mental health care among healthcare professionals by providing these services at no cost. The wellness committee, led by Noah, also introduced a peer-support program. This program connected individuals who were feeling exhausted with others who were currently facing similar challenges. The peer support system provided a valuable space for healthcare professionals to find solace and receive practical advice through exchanging personal stories and empathetic connections.

Appreciating the importance of physical health in overall well-being, Noah and the committee also established regular fitness courses and health tests for the workers. These activities fostered a culture of well-being and strong camaraderie among hospital staff. Noah's work also significantly impacted the hospital's decision to adopt more flexible leave policies, acknowledging the importance of rest and recovery in mitigating burnout. These regulations allowed employees to take time off freely without adverse consequences or judgment. This alteration significantly changed the hospital's perspective on maintaining a healthy equilibrium between work and personal life.

Noah also facilitated town hall meetings with hospital administration and personnel. These meetings offered open discussions about workplace policies, staffing challenges, and other factors contributing to stress and burnout. Establishing this available line of communication between employees and management has enhanced the transparency and responsiveness of the workplace. Noah's initiative had a significant impact. The facility experienced a notable boost in staff morale, resulting in a decrease in turnover rates and an overall improvement in the quality of client care. Noah's approach to addressing burnout has been acknowledged as an exemplary model for other healthcare organisations.

Noah's experience at Mercy Mwongozo Hospital became a captivating narrative of groundbreaking leadership and compassionate advocacy. His endeavours to address burnout in the healthcare field underscored the importance of implementing proactive measures to safeguard the welfare of those who dedicate themselves to the care of others. His work has consistently served as a source of inspiration and guidance, highlighting the crucial importance of a nurturing work environment in maintaining the well-being and effectiveness of healthcare professionals. Noah's campaign highlighted the importance of understanding, working together, and staying determined to establish a healthier, more sustainable workplace.

Noah's efforts to address burnout at Mercy Mwongozo Hospital caught the interest of the broader medical community. Healthcare workers from other hospitals and organisations were eager to learn from his practical strategies. Noah, known for his eagerness to share his knowledge and assist others, initiated webinars and seminars for external healthcare teams. He shared the ideas and practices that had contributed to the success of Mercy Mwongozo's program.

This knowledge exchange led to a collaborative network of healthcare institutions tackling occupational stress and burnout. Noah played a crucial role in this network, advocating for a well-planned approach to tackling the underlying issues contributing to burnout in healthcare environments. The network served as a platform for exchanging resources, methods, and support, amplifying Noah's impact.

Furthermore, Noah shifted his focus towards exploring the role of technology in managing workplace stress. He worked with technology companies to develop applications and resources that help healthcare professionals track their stress levels, organise their schedules, and access mental health resources. These technological advancements provided healthcare professionals with practical tools to manage their well-being.

Appreciating the importance of research in this field, Noah collaborated with academic researchers to study the effects of different strategies on reducing burnout. These studies generated crucial data that improved and reinforced the wellness program's strategies. The study's findings were widely shared, contributing to the growing wealth of knowledge on effectively addressing burnout in healthcare.

Furthermore, Noah's project started significantly influencing policy at both the state and national levels. His campaign, supported by the program's success at Mercy Mwongozo, initiated discussions about potential regulations to improve the mental well-being of healthcare workers. These suggestions encompassed mandatory breaks, limitations on consecutive working hours, and enhanced staffing ratios.

The atmosphere at Mercy Mwongozo was noticeably different. Staff members experienced a greater sense of appreciation and assistance, leading to a more optimistic and cooperative work environment. This adjustment positively impacted both the staff and the quality of client care. The level of client care experienced a significant improvement as healthcare staff experienced reduced stress levels and increased support.

Noah also highlighted the importance of strong leadership in addressing burnout. He facilitated leadership training sessions focused on fostering empathy, effective communication, and promoting the well-being of employees. These courses educated hospital officials on creating a conducive work environment and prioritising mental health and well-being.

Noah's accomplishments in addressing burnout at Mercy Mwongozo Hospital have served as a beacon of hope and a blueprint for other healthcare institutions grappling with similar challenges. His journey exemplified the power of an individual's dedication to ignite significant transformation, resulting in a work environment that promotes the well-being and sustainability of healthcare professionals.

Noah's dedication to tackling worker stress and burnout extended beyond Mercy Mwongozo, catalysing a widespread shift towards a more empathetic and nurturing healthcare system. His endeavours highlighted the importance of taking proactive steps to support the mental well-being of healthcare professionals, guaranteeing they are equipped with the necessary resources and conducive work settings to thrive in their challenging roles. Noah's initiative demonstrated the importance of understanding, creativity, and collaboration in creating a nurturing environment for those dedicated to the well-being of others.

As Noah's projects gained recognition, their influence extended beyond the local healthcare community. The program's achievements at Mercy Mwongozo Hospital catalysed other sectors to adopt a similar approach to addressing job stress and burnout. Noah's approach to resolving these challenges was regarded as exemplary for fostering healthier work environments across various professional disciplines.

Noah's contributions as a leader and advocate in this field led to developing a series of publications and materials detailing the successful strategies and methods employed at Mercy Mwongozo. These tools were widely shared, guiding other organisations interested in implementing similar programs. The papers explored various subjects, from implementing peer support systems to integrating wellness into organizational policies.

In addition to these resources, Noah started collaborating with institutions to incorporate wellness and stress management into their healthcare programs. He emphasised the importance of equipping future healthcare professionals with stress management techniques and prioritising burnout prevention as essential for cultivating a sustainable healthcare workforce. These educational programs highlighted the importance of caring for oneself, being resilient, and seeking assistance when needed.

The conversation surrounding working stress and burnout significantly modified healthcare professionals' training and evaluation methods. Noah's dedication to his cause led to a shift in focus, recognising the importance of clinical skills and the ability to manage personal well-being effectively. This transition was crucial in ensuring that healthcare personnel were technically qualified and emotionally and mentally prepared for the job's demands.

In addition, the program's success led to the establishment of a national conference focused on promoting the well-being of healthcare workers. Noah was crucial in convening healthcare professionals, administrators, policymakers, and mental health experts for this meeting. The conference offered a platform for participants to exchange their experiences, ideas, and innovations regarding improving healthcare worker well-being.

Noah's efforts have led to increased funding for research on the stress and burnout experienced by healthcare workers. This study explores the underlying factors contributing to burnout and effective interventions that can lead to successful solutions for healthcare personnel. The culture shifts towards valuing the welfare of employees at Mercy Mwongozo Hospital flourished. The hospital was frequently recognised as an outstanding example of healthcare employee well-being, drawing in healthcare workers who appreciated a nurturing work environment.

Noah's experience addressing workplace stress and burnout at Mercy Mwongozo Hospital evolved into a tale of transformation, innovation, and advocacy. His unwavering commitment to advancing the welfare of healthcare workers went far beyond the confines of the hospital, leaving a lasting impact on policy, education, and practice across the entire healthcare system. Noah's dedication and guidance in tackling workplace stress and burnout were a powerful testament to supporting those who provide care, leading to a more robust and efficient healthcare system.

Noah's idea ignited a burgeoning movement to enhance the sustainability and supportiveness of healthcare workers' working environments. As the program progressed, its focus expanded to encompass direct care workers and individuals in administrative and support roles within the hospital setting. This comprehensive approach acknowledges the valuable contributions of all individuals in the healthcare setting towards client care and, therefore, emphasises the importance of providing support to manage workplace stress.

Noah was invited to participate in national policy talks due to the program's success. He worked alongside healthcare executives and lawmakers to advocate for legislation prioritising healthcare workers' well-being. His keen insights contributed to formulating policies that mandated routine mental health assessments, adequate staffing, and the implementation of wellness initiatives in healthcare establishments.

In addition to these policy reforms, Noah focused on creating a sustainable paradigm for the program. He established a wellness department at Mercy Mwongozo Hospital, with dedicated professionals focused on maintaining and enhancing the program. This department has become a valuable resource for employees seeking support, offering various services, including individual counselling sessions, group courses, and designated relaxation areas.

Noah's endeavours also led to the establishment of a mentorship program to support healthcare professionals in overcoming the challenges of their profession. Experienced staff members guided and supported newer employees, helping them build resilience and adjust to the challenging healthcare environment. This mentorship program alleviated stress and burnout within the hospital and fostered a culture of collaboration and mutual support.

In addition, Noah tried to address burnout by implementing activities that acknowledged and appreciated the dedication of healthcare personnel. To recognise the commitment and accomplishments of its employees, the hospital initiated a series of regular appreciation gatherings and award ceremonies. These instances are essential reminders of the value and impact of healthcare professionals' work.

Noah's concept started replicating in healthcare institutions nationwide and even worldwide as news of the program's achievements circulated. Healthcare leaders from various countries gathered at Mercy Mwongozo Hospital to learn about the program and its implementation. Noah's approach to managing professional stress and burnout rapidly became the benchmark for promoting wellness among healthcare workers.

Noah's story of conquering professional stress and burnout at Mercy Mwongozo Hospital became a beacon of hope, resilience, and personal growth. The study highlighted the significant impact of a comprehensive wellness program on the health and well-being of healthcare professionals. Noah's insightful perspective in this field has consistently motivated and propelled efforts to create a healthcare environment that is more compassionate and supportive. It aims to acknowledge and address the needs of individuals who dedicate their lives to providing care for others. Noah's efforts to manage workplace stress and burnout showcased the importance of understanding, practical guidance, and creative thinking in cultivating a positive work environment and, consequently, a more robust society.

CHAPTER 21

Medicare for All

S ophia, a healthcare specialist at Mercy Mwongozo Hospital, discovered a pressing problem beyond the hospital's boundaries: a shortage of healthcare availability in marginalised regions. She embarked on a mission to tackle this dilemma directly, driven by a deep commitment to fairness and a passion for equal access to healthcare.

She began by delving into thorough research to gain a deeper understanding of the healthcare challenges faced by these communities. She conducted focus groups and surveys, engaging with marginalised population members to understand their experiences and concerns. This study revealed a complex network of challenges, including economic considerations, cultural misinterpretations, and inadequate healthcare infrastructure in these areas.

Once she gained this insight, Sophia diligently started crafting a comprehensive strategy to address these challenges. She began advocating for mobile health clinics that could reach underserved communities and offer essential medical treatments. These clinics were equipped to provide a wide range of services, from regular health check-ups to specialised medical care.

Sophia forged partnerships with community leaders and organisations alongside the mobile clinics. She emphasised that establishing trust and fostering understanding within these communities was crucial for any healthcare initiative's success. These collaborations helped tailor healthcare services to the unique needs of each community, ensuring they were culturally sensitive and easily accessible.

Sophia also focused on educational and outreach initiatives. She organised health education sessions at community centres, schools, and religious institutions. These programs were designed to enhance public understanding of health issues, promote preventive measures, and provide information on healthcare resources. She ensured that instructional materials were available in multiple languages to broaden their accessibility.

Sophia worked alongside local and state government agencies to enhance healthcare funding in marginalised communities, aiming to eliminate economic obstacles to accessing healthcare. She advocated for legislation offering financial assistance to individuals unable to afford healthcare, thereby reducing the economic burden on these vulnerable populations.

Sophia was dedicated to educating and empowering community health professionals and helping them understand the importance of sustainable healthcare solutions. These workers were crucial in providing healthcare and education within their communities. They acted as intermediaries between healthcare providers and community members, building trust and enabling effective communication.

Sophia's hard work began to yield results. Mobile health clinics were highly regarded, and there was a noticeable rise in healthcare utilisation in their communities. Education and outreach initiatives have enhanced comprehension of health matters and the importance of preventive care, resulting in the overall enhancement of community health.

Sophia's work in addressing healthcare access in marginalised groups is highly impactful. Her holistic approach provided high-quality healthcare and advocated a more equitable healthcare system. Her narrative evolved into a tale of empathy, resolve, and resourcefulness in the battle against disparities in healthcare. Sophia's campaign has consistently motivated and guided, highlighting the crucial role of healthcare professionals in championing and implementing solutions for universal healthcare. Her work exemplified a strong belief in the importance of equal access to healthcare for all, regardless of their background, emphasising the fundamental right to a healthy life.

Sophia's efforts to provide healthcare to underserved regions gained momentum as her work gained recognition and support from more individuals. Her approach extended beyond mere medical services to creating a sustainable healthcare model that could be replicated in different areas.

Sophia's program achieved a significant milestone by establishing community health centres in areas that lacked access to healthcare services. These centres have become essential community resources, offering medical care, health education, and preventive programs. The centres were staffed with highly knowledgeable healthcare professionals with extensive training to address the community's unique health needs.

Sophia was deeply engrossed in exploring digital health initiatives as she sought sustainable healthcare solutions. She dedicated her efforts to developing telehealth services that enabled remote consultations and follow-ups, thereby increasing the accessibility of healthcare for individuals unable to visit a clinic. These digital technologies have played a crucial role in bridging the healthcare access gap, particularly for clients with chronic diseases who require consistent monitoring.

Sophia's dedication to ensuring fairness in healthcare has also motivated her to advocate for improved access to mental health treatment in underserved regions. She acknowledged the often-overlooked importance of mental health in these settings and advocated for the integration of mental health care into existing healthcare programs. She implemented programs to educate community health workers in fundamental mental health treatment and created networks for referring individuals to specialised therapy.

Sophia also understood the importance of addressing the social factors that influence health. She collaborated with community organisations to tackle important issues like housing, nutrition, and education, which are vital to overall health and well-being. Sophia's program improved immediate health outcomes and addressed significant challenges to promote long-term community health and prosperity.

Sophia's projects' success started inspiring similar programs in other locations. Her innovative, all-encompassing healthcare program became a model for addressing healthcare disparities. Healthcare experts from various regions within and outside the country started visiting Sophia's programs to acquire knowledge and implement them in their communities.

Sophia's experience at Mercy Mwongozo Hospital, tackling healthcare access in marginalised communities, evolved into an inspiring tale of hope and change. It was an impressive demonstration of how healthcare workers can drive change and enhance public health. Sophia's work has been a constant source of inspiration and guidance, showcasing the profound impact of compassionate care, community involvement, and steadfast advocacy in creating a more equitable healthcare system. Her endeavours highlighted the crucial contribution of healthcare professionals in expanding care beyond the confines of medical facilities, guaranteeing that healthcare is accessible to all segments of society, especially those who require it the most.

Sophia's work in marginalised communities centred on addressing immediate healthcare needs and promoting long-term health resilience. She implemented community health education programs that empowered individuals to effectively manage common health concerns and make well-informed decisions regarding their health. These programs equipped residents with the necessary skills and knowledge to participate actively in their health and well-being.

Sophia implemented screening programs for various health concerns, acknowledging the importance of early intervention. These tests played a crucial role in identifying and treating illnesses, leading to significant advancements in health outcomes. The success of these screenings highlighted the importance of proactive healthcare and its impact on reducing the disease burden in marginalised communities.

Sophia focused on catering to the unique healthcare needs of vulnerable individuals in these communities, including older people, children, and those with disabilities, as she strived to offer holistic care. She tailored healthcare services to meet the unique needs of each population, ensuring they received the necessary care and attention.

Sophia's work had a profound influence that extended beyond physical well-being. Her initiatives fostered a strong sense of camaraderie and collaboration among the residents. People started coming together to support each other in health and community life.

This strengthening of community bonds showcased the wide-ranging impact of healthcare initiatives beyond mere medical care.

Sophia was dedicated to securing funding and resources to support the ongoing growth of her initiatives. She formed partnerships with non-governmental organisations (NGOs), government agencies, and corporate organisations to raise awareness about the healthcare needs of marginalised groups and garner support for her initiatives. Her skill in uniting individuals from various backgrounds towards a common goal was crucial in ensuring the effectiveness and endurance of her initiatives.

Sophia was committed to analysing and adapting her techniques as her programs constantly evolved. She collected health outcomes and community input information to refine and enhance her programs. This unwavering commitment to continual improvement ensured that her programs stayed effective and adaptable to the community's evolving needs.

Sophia's perspective on healthcare in underserved communities transformed into a model of community involvement and comprehensive care. Her work showcased the profound influence that healthcare professionals can wield when they venture beyond conventional healthcare environments and engage with communities at the grassroots level.

During her time at Mercy Mwongozo Hospital and in the community, she showcased the crucial role of healthcare professionals in addressing healthcare disparities. Sophia's work has consistently served as a source of inspiration and guidance, drawing attention to the vital need for fair healthcare access and emphasising the responsibility of healthcare providers in advocating for and enacting meaningful transformations.

Sophia's commitment to tackling healthcare access in marginalised groups demonstrates a strong belief in the importance of healthcare as a fundamental human right. Her actions showcased the profound impact that committed healthcare professionals can have on the lives of individuals often overlooked by the conventional healthcare system. Her research emphasised the importance of healthcare models prioritising inclusivity, cultural sensitivity, and community engagement, aiming to provide quality treatment for all individuals regardless of socioeconomic status.

Sophia's work in marginalised communities highlighted the interconnectedness of health and social well-being. She collaborated with social service organisations to tackle broader health factors like stable housing, access to nutritious food, and educational opportunities. Sophia's programs enhanced these communities' health outcomes and overall quality of life by addressing their fundamental needs.

Her thorough approach captured the attention of health policymakers and community leaders, leading to the development of more integrated community health projects. Sophia advocated for policies that acknowledged and tackled the social factors influencing health, highlighting the need for a holistic approach to achieving true healthcare fairness.

Sophia started utilising digital platforms to educate and engage the community in her continuous effort to expand the accessibility of healthcare services. She developed online health resources and virtual workshops to enhance the accessibility of health education. These digital technologies proved advantageous in connecting with younger demographics and in areas with limited physical healthcare resources.

Sophia recognised the importance of mental health on overall well-being and therefore incorporated mental health services into her community health programs. She emphasised the importance of integrating mental health care with physical health, recognising it as a crucial aspect of comprehensive healthcare. This integration helped to eliminate the negative perception surrounding mental health in these communities.

Sophia's work also focused on fostering local expertise and skills. She educated community members to become advocates and educators, creating a sustainable model for health and well-being. Sophia's remarkable achievement was empowering individuals within the community, guaranteeing health initiatives' long-term viability and adaptability.

The effectiveness of her programs led to a notable increase in community trust and engagement with healthcare services. Individuals who had previously hesitated to seek medical care started to come forward, confident that they would receive respectful and considerate treatment tailored to their needs.

Sophia's experience at Mercy Mwongozo Hospital and beyond tackling healthcare access in marginalised areas was a tale of empowerment, teamwork, and lasting change. Her work showcased the profound impact that healthcare professionals can make by expanding their care beyond conventional settings and reaching out to communities.

Her endeavours remained a source of inspiration and impact, serving as a paradigm for effectively addressing disparities in healthcare. Sophia's work emphasised the critical role of healthcare professionals in advocating for and implementing inclusive healthcare solutions that address the needs of all community members. Her actions demonstrated a solid commitment to achieving universal healthcare beyond mere ideals. She approached this goal with unwavering dedication, resourcefulness, and a deep understanding of the diverse needs of communities.

Sophia's contribution to transforming community healthcare gained recognition as a paradigm for comprehensive and all-encompassing health approaches. Her research demonstrated that successful healthcare involves more than simply treating diseases; it consists of understanding and addressing the environment in which humans reside.

Sophia prioritised sustainability as her activities expanded. She put in much effort to ensure the long-term sustainability of the progress made in these communities. Her main focus was on educating the next generation to achieve this goal. Sophia initiated health and wellness programs at nearby schools, imparting knowledge to children about nutrition, physical activity, and emotional well-being. These programs aim to cultivate positive habits in children from an early age, laying the foundation for a healthier future.

Sophia also dedicated her efforts to establishing a network of community health advocates. These individuals have undergone training to identify health concerns within their communities and offer support in accessing necessary resources. This network played a crucial role in preserving the significance of her work by fostering a sense of community engagement in the upkeep of their own and their neighbours' well-being.

Sophia diligently arranged frequent training courses for healthcare providers serving marginalised communities, fully understanding the importance of ongoing medical education. These workshops focused on enhancing cultural competency, staying updated with the latest medical techniques, and finding practical solutions for addressing social determinants of health. Sophia played a crucial role in improving the standard of care in these communities by ensuring that healthcare providers were well-prepared and knowledgeable.

Sophia's dedication to healthcare equity motivated her to advocate for more comprehensive policy reforms. She worked closely with local and national policymakers to address and resolve challenges that hindered healthcare access, including transportation issues, insurance coverage gaps, and language barriers. She played a crucial role in shaping a more comprehensive healthcare policy through her advocacy efforts, ensuring that marginalised communities have improved access to essential healthcare services.

Sophia's community healthcare programs achieved remarkable success, garnering recognition from prominent international health organisations. Her community engagement and comprehensive treatment method were adopted in similar programs worldwide, impacting global health initiatives.

Sophia's journey at Mercy Mwongozo Hospital and beyond, revolutionising healthcare in marginalised communities, emerged as a tale of inspiration and enduring change. Her research showcased the power of a comprehensive, community-focused strategy in healthcare and its potential to address health disparities.

Her tireless dedication is a source of inspiration and guidance, highlighting the pivotal role of healthcare professionals in driving positive change and making significant contributions to public health. Sophia's projects showcased the idea of creating a healthcare system that is fair, inclusive, and attentive to the needs of everyone in society through passion, creativity, and a strong understanding of community needs. Her work exemplified a commitment to creating a society where everyone can obtain the necessary healthcare regardless of their financial situation to lead a fulfilling and well-rounded life.

CHAPTER 22

Emma's Personal Touch

Emma, a nurse at Mercy Mwongozo Hospital, faced a new challenge: maintaining a personal connection in an ever-evolving digital healthcare environment. She embarked on a mission to find the perfect equilibrium between harnessing technological advancements and preserving the compassionate, empathetic nature at the core of nursing. She began by evaluating the current utilisation of technology in client care at the hospital. Emma conducted surveys and interviews with healthcare personnel and clients to understand how technology impacted their experiences. She carefully assessed the practicality and influence of each tool on the interaction between clients and carers, ranging from electronic health records to telemedicine.

Emma utilised this information to develop a comprehensive training program for hospital staff. She aimed to educate her colleagues on integrating technology as a complement to, rather than a substitute for, conventional nursing practices. The program included sessions on enhancing communication through digital platforms, maintaining empathy in virtual consultations, and utilising technology to customise client care. Emma also initiated a series of workshops for clients to educate them about digital health literacy. She understood that for technology to be an effective tool in healthcare, it was crucial for individuals to feel comfortable with it and have the necessary skills to utilise it. These courses educated individuals on using different healthcare technologies, empowering them to engage in their care actively.

Emma was dedicated to incorporating technology to enhance client engagement and comfort while maintaining the personal aspect of healthcare. She strongly supported implementing user-friendly apps that allowed for convenient monitoring of health indicators and effortless communication with medical professionals. These technologies helped clients gain a sense of empowerment over their health and fostered a stronger connection with their healthcare providers.

Appreciating the immense possibilities of artificial intelligence and machine learning in enhancing client outcomes, Emma worked with the hospital's IT team to develop AI tools that complemented the nursing staff rather than overshadowed them. AI-powered diagnostic assistance systems and predictive analytics for client care were among the tools that provided valuable insights while enabling nurses to stay at the forefront of decision-making. Emma was dedicated to safeguarding client privacy and confidentiality, ensuring technology would not compromise these essential aspects. She collaborated with the hospital's IT department to enhance data security and guided staff on effective methods for managing client information in the digital age.

Emma's work had a profound impact. Clients at Mercy Mwongozo Hospital expressed a heightened sense of involvement and contentment with their care, even in cases where technology played a significant role. The staff found a renewed sense of purpose by embracing technology to enhance their caregiving, fostering a closer connection with their clients.

Emma's experience at Mercy Mwongozo Hospital navigating the intersection of technology and personal care unfolded as a tale of ingenuity, compassion, and purposeful blending. Her work highlighted the importance of embracing technological advancements while upholding the fundamental principles of nursing care. Emma's dedication remains a source of inspiration and guidance, highlighting the crucial role of healthcare professionals in shaping the future of client care. This future envisions a harmonious blend of technology and human interaction, delivering compassionate, streamlined, and individualised care.

Emma's innovative approach to merging technology and personal care started to make waves in the broader healthcare community. She championed a client-centred approach to healthcare technology utilisation, sharing her insights at numerous industry conferences and seminars. Her message was clear: technology should enhance, rather than substitute, the human elements of empathy, compassion, and understanding in client care.

Emma implemented a feedback mechanism to allow clients to share their experiences using technology in their care as part of her ongoing efforts at Mercy Mwongozo Hospital. This input offered valuable insights that helped refine the balance between digital and personal care. It ensured that the hospital's utilisation of technology always aligned with the client's needs and preferences. Emma recognised the importance of emotional intelligence in healthcare. She facilitated training workshops for healthcare professionals to enhance their abilities. This training helped staff effectively convey empathy and compassion through digital communication.

Emma also collaborated with technology developers, healthcare professionals, and clients. The objective was to develop user-friendly healthcare technologies that promoted a positive client-caregiver dynamic. This collaborative design method ensured that new technologies were created with a comprehensive understanding of the requirements of end users.

Emma's work had a significant effect on the satisfaction and engagement of both clients and healthcare staff. Clients expressed a heightened sense of involvement and empowerment in their healthcare experiences. At the same time, staff members found greater satisfaction in their professions, all thanks to the implementation of technology that enhanced operations and offered valuable insights into client care. Emma's work at Mercy Mwongozo Hospital exemplified a harmonious blend of cutting-edge technology and empathetic client care, resulting in a progressive and compassionate healthcare narrative. Her narrative showcased the profound impact of leveraging technology in healthcare, leading to more meaningful and productive client interactions.

Emma's dedication to finding a harmonious balance between technology and personal care is a source of inspiration and guidance for others. She has set a remarkable example for healthcare professionals adapting to the evolving medical technology landscape. Her work showcased the power of technology in enhancing healthcare quality while keeping the client at the forefront as a unique individual with specific needs and experiences. Emma's endeavours demonstrated that, within the realm of healthcare, despite the constant progress of technology, the human element remained indispensable and essential.

Emma's dedication to blending technology with personal care evolved, becoming a defining characteristic of her healthcare approach. She understood the importance of staying informed and flexible in the ever-changing field of medical technology. Her goal was to use technology to enhance the quality of care while still maintaining the essential human connection needed for healing.

Emma thoroughly explored the possibilities of virtual reality (VR) and augmented reality (AR) in client education and rehabilitation as a natural extension of her ongoing efforts. These virtual experiences can significantly enhance clients' understanding of their diseases and treatments. VR simulations, for instance, were used to help clients visualise and understand their medical procedures, reducing anxiety and improving client preparedness.

Emma quickly acknowledged the possibilities of wearable technology in monitoring client health. She strongly supported implementing technologies that could provide clients and healthcare practitioners with up-to-date health data. These wearables helped in the early detection of potential health issues and encouraged proactive healthcare management.

Her focus on technology, however, was always complemented by a strong desire to maintain a personal connection. Emma ensured that personal follow-ups accompanied every technology interaction. She educated her team on the value of using technology to enhance client interactions, emphasising the importance of human engagement. Emma's innovative approach also involved developing a client portal, enabling seamless communication between clients and their healthcare providers. Clients could access their medical records, communicate with their healthcare team, and receive personalised health recommendations and reminders via this portal. It empowered clients to participate actively in their healthcare journey, fostering a collaborative partnership between clients and doctors.

Emma was deeply engrossed in examining the ethical implications of healthcare technology, striving to find the perfect equilibrium between technological advancements and personalised care. She organised discussions and debates on data protection, informed consent in the digital age, and the ethical use of artificial intelligence in healthcare. These discussions raised awareness and fostered a culture of moral responsibility in using technology at Mercy Mwongozo Hospital.

The success of Emma's activities garnered attention from healthcare organisations and technology entrepreneurs. She was invited to participate in projects to create cutting-edge healthcare technology that prioritises clients' needs and adheres to ethical standards. These collaborations offered opportunities to prioritise healthcare practitioners' and clients' perspectives and requirements in technological innovation in healthcare.

Emma's work also influenced the hospital staff. Integrating technology in client care has enhanced efficiency and streamlined processes, alleviating the workload and enabling healthcare providers to dedicate more time to direct client care. This change resulted in increased employee job satisfaction and a work atmosphere that is more positive and focused on client care.

Emma's work at Mercy Mwongozo Hospital to balance technology and personal care became a tale of groundbreaking and empathetic treatment. Her path showcased the profound impact of utilising technology thoughtfully and ethically in healthcare settings.

Emma's dedication has consistently motivated and directed, showcasing a future of cutting-edge healthcare while deeply rooted in empathy and comprehension. Her work highlighted the crucial impact of healthcare professionals on integrating technology in client care, guaranteeing that advancements in medical technology lead to improved client experiences and outcomes. Emma's work highlighted the enduring importance of the human touch in healthcare, even in the face of technological progress. Emma's journey at Mercy Mwongozo Hospital in integrating technology with personal care continued to grow, resulting in a healthcare approach that was both forward-thinking and deeply compassionate. Her work started to make a difference not just in the operations of her hospital but also in the broader conversation about the use of technology in healthcare.

Emma's primary focus revolved around leveraging data analytics to enhance client care. She worked alongside a team of data scientists to analyse client data, aiming to uncover patterns and trends that could lead to more personalised and effective treatment approaches. However, Emma ensured that these insights were consistently utilised to enhance, rather than supplant, the healthcare team's judgment and experience. She supported a well-rounded approach that combined data-driven insights with human intuition.

Emma developed a system to gather client feedback on technology usage, demonstrating her commitment to prioritising the client experience in healthcare. This approach enabled clients to share their experiences and comments directly, ensuring that technology was always utilised in alignment with their needs and comfort. This feedback was instrumental in consistently enhancing the utilisation of technology in client care.

Emma recognised the importance of emotional support in healing and recovery. She was at the forefront of utilising technology to connect clients with their loved ones, especially when in-person visits were not feasible. Virtual visitation systems were implemented, enabling clients to stay in touch with their loved ones and maintain crucial emotional bonds.

Emma's work also included developing training programs for healthcare organisations looking to incorporate technology into their client care procedures. These programs shared valuable insights, challenges, and knowledge gained, helping other healthcare providers overcome obstacles in implementing technology to enhance client care.

Emma's work had a profound influence beyond the immediate advantages of improved client care and efficiency. It also focused on enhancing the client-caregiver interaction. Healthcare providers have streamlined their regular tasks through technology, allowing them to dedicate more time to building meaningful client relationships. This has resulted in the development of crucial bonds of trust and empathy in healthcare.

Emma's story at Mercy Mwongozo Hospital exemplifies the transformative power of technology in healthcare when applied with wisdom and compassion. Her experience showcased the potential of technology to enhance the human elements of healthcare, resulting in greater effectiveness, efficiency, and compassion.

Emma's project has continued to captivate and shape, paving the path for a future where healthcare technology seamlessly integrates with a personal touch. Her research emphasised the crucial role of healthcare professionals in guiding technology into client care, guaranteeing that advancements in medical technology are consistently rooted in the core principles of compassion, empathy, and client-centred care. Emma's dedication is evident in her pursuit of a healthcare system that prioritises human connection and aims to improve the client experience.

Emma's efforts in merging technology and personal care have led to the development of a comprehensive program to enhance client education and engagement. She developed interactive digital platforms that empower clients to learn about their health conditions, explore treatment options, and adopt wellness strategies. These platforms were designed to focus on ease of use and accessibility, empowering clients to engage actively in their healthcare journey. Emma ensured that various instructional materials were accessible in multiple languages and formats, catering to different learning styles and preferences and acknowledging clients' diverse needs. She also incorporated features that encouraged clients to inquire and receive tailored responses, enhancing their comprehension and involvement in healthcare.

Emma explored the potential of remote monitoring systems as she sought to leverage technology for improved client care. These systems allowed chronically ill clients to be monitored at home, reducing the necessity for frequent hospital visits. Healthcare providers utilise the data gathered by these platforms to make well-informed treatment and care decisions. This approach provided clients convenience and ensured ongoing treatment and monitoring, improving health results.

Emma's work has also led to collaboration with technology companies to create health solutions that prioritise clients' needs. These apps offered a range of features, including medication reminders, health tracking, and virtual consultations. Emma ensured that these applications were tailored to meet users' needs by involving clients and healthcare providers in the development process, resulting in increased effectiveness and widespread adoption.

Emma also coordinated community outreach programs to educate the Mwongozo population about the advantages and uses of healthcare technology. These programs aimed to narrow the digital divide and guarantee equal access to digital health technologies for individuals from diverse backgrounds. This initiative successfully addressed the needs of older individuals and marginalised communities, who often face obstacles in accessing digital healthcare services.

Emma's endeavours had a profound impact at Mercy Mwongozo Hospital and beyond. Clients reported increased satisfaction with their care, while healthcare workers experienced a renewed sense of purpose and efficiency. The hospital became a prime example for other institutions seeking to incorporate client-centred technology into healthcare.

Emma's remarkable journey of blending technology with human care is a captivating tale of innovation, compassion, and exceptional guidance. Through her diligent work, there was a notable transformation in the delivery and perception of healthcare. This showcased the immense impact that technology, when paired with a deep comprehension of client needs, can have on enhancing the quality and overall care experience. Emma's endeavours have consistently sparked inspiration and exerted a profound impact on the trajectory of healthcare, showcasing the seamless integration of technology and human connection. Her work highlighted the critical role of healthcare professionals in shaping client care, utilising technology to enhance client outcomes and foster a solid caregiver-client bond. Emma's journey showcased a commitment to a healthcare system that is highly advanced in technology, genuinely compassionate, and focused on the client's needs.

CHAPTER 23

David's Global Perspective

D avid, a respected individual at Mercy Mwongozo Hospital for his expertise and empathetic approach to healthcare, expanded his perspectives to tackle global health concerns. His journey started when he received an invitation to participate in an international health program focused on enhancing healthcare access and quality in underserved regions across the globe. His deep engagement in the endeavour showcases his broad range of experiences and unwavering commitment to achieving fairness in healthcare. David was tasked with leading a team of healthcare specialists to develop strategies for tackling urgent global health issues, including infectious diseases, hunger, and limited access to healthcare services.

David and his team embarked on an extensive study to gain a deeper understanding of the distinct healthcare needs of various communities across the globe. This study necessitated a strong partnership with local healthcare providers, community leaders, and clients to gain a comprehensive understanding of the challenges they faced. The findings obtained from this research were crucial in establishing culturally sensitive and sustainable therapies.

David played a crucial role in establishing mobile healthcare clinics, one of his main initiatives. These clinics were set to extend their reach to remote and underserved regions, providing essential medical services where necessary. These mobile clinics, equipped with the required medical supplies and staffed by skilled healthcare professionals, significantly improved healthcare accessibility in these communities. David focused on educating and providing training programs for local healthcare workers, alongside delivering direct healthcare treatment. He was convinced that imparting knowledge and skills to local populations was crucial for achieving lasting transformation. The training programs covered various topics, including primary healthcare practices and more specialised medical treatments.

David played a crucial role in establishing partnerships with both local and international organisations. These collaborations were critical to acquiring the resources and support necessary for the initiative's success. They also fostered the sharing of knowledge and best practices, amplifying the health initiative's impact. David also advocated integrating technology to enhance healthcare delivery in these global communities. He focused on implementing telehealth services, which allowed for remote consultations and support, overcoming geographical barriers, and requiring more local healthcare expertise.

David's impact on the global health campaign was substantial. Communities that previously faced challenges in accessing primary healthcare services started to observe improvements in health outcomes and overall well-being. The success stories from these areas are a testament to the effectiveness of David and his team's activities.

David's involvement in the global health project exemplified a remarkable display of international cooperation, creativity, and empathy. His work highlighted the crucial role of healthcare professionals in addressing global health disparities. David's work has been a source of inspiration and guidance, shedding light on a more equitable and healthier society where everyone, regardless of location, can receive high-quality treatment. His involvement in the global health effort highlighted the significant impact committed and skilled healthcare professionals could make, improving lives and communities through exceptional healthcare and innovation.

David's participation in the global health project developed as he encountered fresh challenges and explored innovative solutions to intricate health issues. One of his notable achievements was in illness prevention and control. David and his team developed community-based programs aimed at preventing common diseases. These initiatives included vaccination campaigns, efforts to improve sanitation, and public health education. These programs played a crucial role in decreasing the occurrence of infectious diseases in vulnerable regions.

David implemented targeted healthcare programs focused on women's health, recognising women's crucial contribution to the well-being of their families and communities. These initiatives focused on important issues like maternal and reproductive health and ensuring access to family planning services. By empowering women with information and healthcare services, these initiatives improved women's health and positively impacted the community's overall health.

David highlighted the importance of developing local healthcare capabilities to offer long-term solutions. He advocated for establishing training centres to provide continuous education and training to healthcare providers in the local community. These centres were instrumental in fostering the growth of healthcare infrastructure in disadvantaged regions, guaranteeing a reliable presence of skilled healthcare professionals for the communities.

David's approach to global health strategy focused on tackling the underlying factors that influence people's health. He prioritised projects that improved access to clean water, nutrition, and education, recognising the strong connection between these factors and health outcomes. These projects provided immediate benefits and laid the foundation for long-term improvements in the health of these communities.

David's global health initiative garnered widespread recognition and backing worldwide. Funding agencies and international health organisations saw the value in expanding their investments in the programs, which allowed them to have a greater reach and make a more significant impact. David's exceptional leadership in these programs showcases the power of a holistic, cooperative approach to addressing global health concerns. David maintained a deep connection to his roots as a healthcare provider at Mercy Mwongozo Hospital throughout his journey. He often discussed his international experiences with his colleagues, offering valuable perspectives and motivating them to think about the broader significance of their work. His narratives and encounters sparked admiration among numerous individuals at the hospital, fostering a culture of worldwide health awareness and accountability.

David's participation in the global health project unfolded as a tale of hope, strength, and international solidarity. His actions showcased the power of dedicated healthcare professionals to impact the world significantly, irrespective of borders or cultural challenges. David's project has consistently served as a source of inspiration and guidance, highlighting the vital importance of healthcare professionals in shaping global health outcomes and advocating for a more equitable and healthier world. His journey exemplified a commitment to a global perspective on healthcare, ensuring that every person, no matter where they are, can enjoy wellness. David's impact on the worldwide health initiative extended beyond specific projects or programs. His work helped shape a broader narrative in international health policy and strategy. Appreciating his knowledge and achievements, global health organisations started to approach David for his contribution to formulating health policies that could be implemented in diverse environments across the globe.

David's primary focus revolved around enhancing healthcare systems, especially in regions susceptible to health emergencies like epidemics or natural disasters. He guided the design of emergency response methods and the construction of robust health infrastructure capable of withstanding similar crises, drawing from his wealth of experience. His proposals highlighted the importance of quick action and long-term planning in sustaining healthcare services during and after emergencies.

David also became a passionate advocate for mental health, which is sometimes overlooked in global health debates. He initiated mental health programs that provided support not only to clients but also to healthcare personnel who faced high levels of stress in challenging circumstances. His research highlighted the interconnectedness of physical and mental well-being and the importance of holistic treatment that addresses both aspects.

David's endeavours also included tackling persistent health conditions, which were increasingly widespread worldwide. He collaborated with experts to develop community-based disease prevention and management programs, including diabetes and hypertension. These programs included initiatives focused on improving lifestyle choices, routine health assessments, and fostering community among clients and their families.

David strongly emphasised fostering connections and working together to improve global health. He encouraged the collaboration of non-governmental organisations, government agencies, healthcare providers, and community organisations to tackle complex health concerns through a unified approach. These collaborations were crucial in bringing together resources, exchanging knowledge, and implementing extensive health programs.

Another crucial aspect of David's work was his unwavering commitment to using technology in global health. He was involved in projects that used digital tools for health education, remote diagnostics, and telemedicine. These technological solutions proved highly efficient in remote and underserved areas with limited access to healthcare personnel and facilities.

David embraced a comprehensive approach to global health, considering medical needs and social and environmental factors that impact well-being. He supported initiatives that improved access to clean water, nutritious food, and safe living conditions, recognising their crucial role in promoting good health. Under David's guidance, the global health program produced substantial advantages. Communities that had previously struggled with low health outcomes started to make significant strides in health and well-being. The success of these endeavours showcased David's approach, which combined practical knowledge with strategic analysis.

David's involvement in the global health project became an inspiring tale of growth, collaboration, and innovation. His initiatives showcased the effectiveness of empathetic and intelligent leadership in addressing global health challenges. David's work has consistently motivated and educated individuals globally, showcasing the profound impact that can be achieved when passion, expertise, and a steadfast dedication to fairness and righteousness guide healthcare initiatives.

His project demonstrated the profound influence healthcare practitioners can have on global health, extending far beyond their local communities. David's work emphasised the importance of healthcare professionals in shaping global health outcomes, advocating for a comprehensive, adaptable, and robust global healthcare system. His journey demonstrated a commitment to creating a society where every person, regardless of location or financial status, can obtain the necessary healthcare to lead a fulfilling and healthy life.

David's activities within the global health framework revolutionised healthcare procedures and changed the perspectives of those involved in healthcare delivery. His focus on cultural sensitivity and local engagement in healthcare solutions contributed to a deeper understanding of the diverse healthcare needs. This understanding led to more efficient and empathetic methods of healthcare provision, particularly in areas with various cultural customs and values.

David understood the significance of implementing sustainable approaches in his mission to enhance global health. He worked on projects exploring the relationship between environmental and public health, aiming to understand their interconnectedness better. Among these programs were initiatives to improve sanitation, reduce pollution, and ensure access to clean drinking water. David's efforts contributed to the prevention of various health conditions by focusing on environmental factors and enhancing community resilience and self-sufficiency.

David also mentored and motivated numerous young healthcare professionals who were enthusiastic about global health. He generously shared his experiences and views through lectures, seminars, and mentorship programs. His narratives of challenges and achievements in the field provided valuable insights for individuals aspiring to impact global health. David's guidance played a crucial role in shaping a new generation of healthcare professionals who are passionate about promoting global health equity and well-prepared to make a positive impact. In addition, David's broad outlook prompted him to support allocating more resources towards health research in disadvantaged regions. He was convinced that gaining a comprehensive understanding and efficiently tackling health issues specific to certain areas necessitated conducting research at the local level. This campaign significantly contributed to the global pool of health knowledge by rallying support for constructing research facilities and funding studies in these locations.

David's achievements led to increased global cooperation. His work emphasised the importance of international collaboration in tackling global health issues through sharing knowledge, resources, and skills. These international collaborations led to the development of more robust health systems equipped to address health issues at both local and global levels. The narrative surrounding David's involvement in the worldwide health initiative revolved around dismantling obstacles, connecting disparate groups, and fostering an international network to enhance health outcomes for everyone. His journey showcased the unwavering commitment of healthcare professionals to overcome barriers and achieve significant advancements in global health.

David's project has continued to be a source of inspiration and guidance, shedding light on the crucial role of healthcare professionals in spearheading global health initiatives. His work demonstrates the potential to build a healthier world through commitment, teamwork, and a comprehensive understanding of diverse health needs. David's journey exemplified a solid commitment to creating a future where health equity becomes tangible. This vision was achieved through the collective efforts of passionate individuals and communities across the globe.

David's impact on global health expanded as he explored innovative strategies to tackle the mounting challenges in healthcare. He was fascinated by integrating traditional medicine practices with modern healthcare approaches, especially in regions where conventional medicine was deeply rooted in cultural norms. He worked alongside local healers and doctors to create a harmonious combination of traditional and modern medical practices, providing culturally sensitive and comprehensive healthcare.

This integration improved client outcomes and fostered respect and understanding among diverse medical traditions. It laid the foundation for a healthcare system that embraced and valued various medical knowledge systems. David passionately championed global health justice at various international events alongside his dedicated work in the field. He highlighted the disparities in health between affluent nations and developing countries, advocating for a fairer allocation of healthcare resources and technology. David's campaign highlighted the importance of global health policies that transcend political and economic barriers, focusing on the fundamental right to health.

His efforts also encompassed establishing health programs that specifically addressed the requirements of children and teenagers in disadvantaged regions. Understanding the importance of children's health for the well-being of any community, these programs focused on proactive healthcare, proper nutrition, and addressing common childhood illnesses. They also educated young individuals about health and cleanliness, empowering them to make informed choices for their well-being.

David also acknowledged the increasing global concern regarding noncommunicable diseases (NCDs). He led research efforts focused on studying risk factors for non-communicable diseases, including unhealthy eating habits, lack of exercise, and tobacco consumption. These endeavours contributed to preventing NCDs and offered support and care to individuals already affected by them. The positive health statistics and happy expressions in the communities David collaborated with showcased the effectiveness of his concepts. His work catalysed the development of similar health programs in various locations, contributing to a worldwide effort to enhance health outcomes for everyone.

David's involvement in the global health project became an awe-inspiring tale of empathy, creativity, and determination. His actions showcased the profound global influence that healthcare professionals can have. David's work has consistently motivated and uplifted individuals striving to impact global health positively. His projects showcased the strength of collective effort and universal compassion in addressing global health issues. David's path represented a dedication to a world in which every person, regardless of where they are born, has the opportunity to live a healthy and whole life.

CHAPTER 24

Evolution of Education

Lina, a nurse educator and inventor at Mercy Mwongozo Hospital, embarked on a mission to transform nursing education. She aimed to create a program to stimulate critical thinking while emphasising the importance of hands-on, empathetic client care. This endeavour, however, was met with both resistance and notable advancements.

She began by creating a comprehensive curriculum that combined conventional nursing education with cutting-edge, inventive methods. She desired to incorporate simulation-based learning, inter-professional education, and a more prominent emphasis on mental health and holistic care. Lina thought that nurses should be well-equipped to handle the evolving requirements of contemporary healthcare, thereby requiring a broader range of skills.

Lina faced resistance from her colleagues and institutions in the cities, who needed to be more cautious about straying from the established curriculum. Some individuals expressed apprehension about the potential impact of the new methods on the long-standing emphasis on rigorous medical expertise in nursing education. Lina, however, remained undisturbed. She conducted presentations and workshops to showcase the effectiveness of her proposed methods, illustrating how they could enhance nursing education and, consequently, client care.

Her determination started to yield results over time. Lina experimented with her new approach in several classes, and the outcomes showed great potential. Students in these seminars showcased enhanced academic performance and a profound understanding of client care, empathy, and critical thinking. They demonstrated a high level of proficiency in navigating intricate clinical environments and working effectively with colleagues from various disciplines.

Lina's endeavours were expanded due to her achievements. She developed cultural competency modules to equip nurses with the skills to provide care in a diverse community. She also integrated mental health training into the curriculum, educating future nurses on the importance of mental well-being for themselves and their clients.

Lina's remarkable achievements in her trial programs caught the attention of numerous nursing schools and healthcare institutions, propelling her into the spotlight. She began receiving invitations to speak at conferences and participate in forums discussing the future of nursing education. Her methods, which had previously been met with scepticism, were now praised as one-of-a-kind and essential.

Lina's hard work has led to successful partnerships with healthcare technology companies, enabling nursing students to access simulation tools and virtual reality experiences. These tools offer students practical and immersive learning experiences, equipping them for real-world clinical settings within a secure and supervised environment.

Lina's endeavours had a profound influence that extended far beyond the confines of the classroom. Upon entering the profession, her pupils received high praise for their exceptional abilities and comprehensive approach to client care. Their industry recognised them as pioneers, blending their deep knowledge of technology with a genuine concern for others.

Lina's narrative of academic advancement at Mercy Mwongozo Hospital's nursing school unfolded as a tale of unwavering perseverance, resourcefulness, and unwavering resolve. Her experience showcased the profound impact of education in shaping the future of healthcare. Lina's project has consistently served as a source of inspiration and guidance, highlighting the crucial role of educators in equipping healthcare practitioners with the necessary skills, knowledge, and empathy to tackle contemporary healthcare challenges. Her actions demonstrated a commitment to a progressive, comprehensive, and empathetic approach to nursing education, paving the path for a new wave of nurses ready to impact their clients' lives significantly.

Lina's pedagogical changes gained momentum, and she turned her attention to another crucial aspect of nursing education: nursing students' emotional and psychological well-being. Understanding the demanding nature of the nursing profession, she integrated modules focused on self-care, stress management, and building resilience. These programs were created to equip students with the necessary resources to maintain their mental well-being in a demanding work setting.

Lina's perspective on a more comprehensive nursing education strongly emphasised research and evidence-based practice. She encouraged students to actively engage in research projects and stay current on the latest healthcare trends. This approach fostered a perpetual learning and innovation mindset among students, equipping them to go beyond their caregiving roles and actively contribute to advancing nursing.

Lina also acknowledged the importance of strong leadership skills in the nursing field. She integrated leadership training into the curriculum, equipping students for future leadership roles. This course covered a range of subjects, including team management, effective communication, and decision-making. Lina strongly emphasised the importance of equipping nurses with leadership skills to drive the growth and evolution of the healthcare system.

Lina's achievements led to fruitful partnerships with various healthcare organisations and nursing schools. These collaborations fostered a rich exchange of ideas and resources, enhancing the nursing education program at Mercy Mwongozo Hospital. Lina's innovative approaches established fresh standards in nursing education, impacting the curriculum at institutions beyond her own.

The feedback from Lina's nursing program graduates was highly favourable. Many alums credited the program for their diverse skill set and ability to adapt to clinical contexts. Employers also noted the impressive preparation and professionalism displayed by the program's graduates.

Lina's endeavour to transform nursing education at Mercy Mwongozo Hospital was a tale of vision and lasting impact. Her research highlighted education's crucial role in shaping healthcare professionals' future. Lina's initiative continued to inspire and guide, showcasing nursing education's ability to adapt to changing healthcare needs.

Her initiatives showcased a solid commitment to nurturing skilled healthcare professionals and fostering empathetic, determined, and forward-thinking nursing executives. Lina's work was a powerful testament to the idea that the education of healthcare workers plays a crucial role in shaping the future of healthcare. Her journey showcased the profound influence of cutting-edge educational methods in equipping nurses with the expertise, understanding, and compassion needed to tackle the complexities of contemporary healthcare.

Lina's innovative approach to nursing education captured the interest of global educational and health organisations. Appreciating the worldwide significance of her approaches, she received invitations to share her ideas and strategies at various international conferences, thereby contributing to the shaping of the future of nursing education on a global level. Her approach of combining practical skills, emotional intelligence, and leadership training was seen as a blueprint for developing versatile healthcare professionals who can easily adjust to the evolving demands of the global healthcare industry.

Lina highlighted the significance of interprofessional education in her dedication to achieving excellence in nursing education. She spearheaded innovative training programs that fostered collaboration between nursing students and their counterparts in the medical, pharmacy, and social work fields. These programs promoted a collaborative approach to client care by dismantling barriers between healthcare disciplines. This approach to interprofessional education equips students with the collaborative nature of contemporary healthcare, where effective communication and teamwork play a vital role in delivering top-notch client care.

Lina made a diligent effort to integrate global health concepts into the nursing curriculum. She established exchange programs with nursing schools in different countries, allowing students to experience healthcare systems and practices in diverse cultural and socioeconomic contexts. These experiences broadened the students' understanding, enriching their knowledge of global health concerns and various healthcare delivery techniques.

Another crucial aspect of Lina's work was her unwavering commitment to utilising technology in nursing education. She seamlessly integrated digital tools and online learning platforms into the curriculum to ensure students could use technology in clinical settings. These digital skills were crucial in equipping students for a healthcare environment heavily relying on technology for client care, data administration, and communication.

Lina's educational changes were evident in the enhanced quality of client care for her program graduates. Those who had completed Lina's curriculum showcased clinical competence and exceptional critical thinking, empathy, and adaptability in diverse healthcare environments. Their excellent blend of technical expertise and compassionate care set a groundbreaking benchmark in nursing.

Lina also initiated an ongoing development process for the nursing program. She established feedback loops with current students, alumni, and healthcare businesses to regularly analyse and adjust the curriculum. This process guaranteed that the information provided stayed up-to-date, efficient, and aligned with the latest healthcare trends and requirements.

Lina's work at Mercy Mwongozo Hospital in nursing education transformation is a remarkable tale of creativity, dedication, and wide-ranging impact. Her experience highlighted the crucial role of academics in shaping the future of healthcare professions. Lina's activities inspired and guided others, laying the foundation for a transformative era in nursing education.

Her initiatives demonstrated a solid commitment to cultivating healthcare professionals with clinical expertise and the ability to lead, innovate, and provide compassionate client care in a rapidly evolving healthcare landscape. Lina's work exemplified the power of education in preparing healthcare workers to navigate the complexities and advancements of modern healthcare. Her journey highlighted the vital significance of forward-thinking educational methods in equipping nurses to positively impact healthcare outcomes, client experiences, and the overall improvement of health systems worldwide.

Lina's efforts in revolutionising nursing education began to have a significant influence on the global healthcare community. Her approaches were not only innovative but also focused on meeting the fundamental requirements of modern healthcare. She trained versatile, compassionate, and highly proficient practitioners in multiple domains.

Lina's focus on interprofessional education started to impact the functioning of clinical teams. Graduates of her program fostered a culture of collaboration in their workplaces, effectively communicating and working with experts from various healthcare disciplines. Due to this transformation, healthcare teams have become more unified and skilled in providing thorough and integrated client care.

Her commitment to incorporating global health concepts also had a significant influence. Her exchange students returned with much knowledge and experience, prepared to apply international health concepts in their local practices. This exposure to various healthcare systems and practices fostered the development of nurses with a deep understanding of different cultures and a strong global perspective.

In addition, Lina's focus on technology in nursing education showcased a progressive mindset. She taught students digital skills to be equipped for the present healthcare landscape and upcoming advancements. Her graduates were highly respected for their ability to quickly embrace and apply healthcare technologies, improving client care in efficiency and effectiveness.

The exceptional quality of client care delivered by Lina's program graduates is a clear testament to the effectiveness of her educational reforms. These nurses were highly regarded for their sharp analytical abilities, adeptness in handling complex clinical matters, and unwavering dedication to providing compassionate client care. Their impact went beyond individual client interactions, leading to higher standards of care and increased client satisfaction in the hospitals they served.

Lina's approach to enhancing the nursing curriculum ensured that the education remained adaptable and responsive to the constantly evolving healthcare environment. This approach ensured that the curriculum remained at the forefront of healthcare education, and her program became a benchmark for nursing schools worldwide.

Lina's work at Mercy Mwongozo Hospital to reform nursing education became a captivating story of how forward-thinking and unwavering commitment to excellence can transform a profession. Her journey showcased the profound impact that educators can have on shaping not just their students' intellect but also the future of medical practices. Lina's initiatives laid the foundation for a new era in nursing education, blending technical expertise with compassion and strong leadership skills. This approach equips nurses to go beyond caregiving and become pioneers, influencers, and champions. Her work showed the critical role of education in preparing healthcare workers to tackle the difficulties of a fast-shifting healthcare landscape and have a significant, positive impact on health systems and client care globally.

Lina's forward-thinking approach to nursing education has significantly impacted healthcare policy discussions and the establishment of educational benchmarks. Her remarkable accomplishment at Mercy Mwongozo Hospital has been a blueprint for successful educational reform, sparking meaningful conversations with healthcare education boards and regulatory organisations. She advocated for implementing curriculum reforms on a national and even global level, highlighting the significance of a contemporary approach that aligns with the realities and requirements of modern healthcare.

She also dedicated herself to advancing nursing leadership and mentorship programs. Lina was committed to fostering the growth of future nursing leaders who would drive innovation and excellence in the field. These programs focused on mentorship, strategic thinking, and change management skills, equipping nurses to play vital roles in shaping the future of healthcare.

Lina also started focusing on research in nursing education. She collaborated with academic institutions to research the impact of her educational innovations, offering concrete evidence of their effectiveness. This study was crucial in advocating for broader implementation of her methods as it demonstrated a direct link between her instructional approaches and enhanced client care outcomes. In addition, Lina's efforts started to revolutionise nursing faculty recruitment and training. She highlighted the significance of instructors with clinical competence and a deep understanding of innovative teaching methods. This modification ensured that the faculty could effectively implement the redesigned curriculum while promoting a culture of ongoing learning and development.

Lina's contributions had a significant influence on the broader healthcare community as well. Healthcare professionals who collaborated with graduates of her program observed a notable enhancement in the quality of nursing care. These nurses brought a wide range of skills, a deep understanding of client needs, and a solid ability to think critically, all of which enhanced the effectiveness of the healthcare team. Lina's remarkable impact on nursing education at Mercy Mwongozo Hospital was a testament to her commitment to excellence and ability to think outside the box. Her work showcased the profound impact of passionate educators on a profession, shaping individuals' skills and knowledge and the overall standards and practices of the entire sector.

Lina's activities have continued to inspire and impact others, demonstrating the transformative power of education in educating healthcare workers in a rapidly changing environment. Her research highlighted educators' crucial role in preparing skilled, compassionate, and visionary healthcare professionals. Lina's journey exemplified a commitment to a future where nursing education evolves, pioneers, and takes the lead in producing nurses equipped to address modern healthcare challenges and drive forward positive transformation within the field. Her initiatives emphasised the crucial role of cutting-edge educational methods in cultivating a healthcare workforce that can deliver exceptional client care and make substantial contributions to the global enhancement of health systems.

CHAPTER 25

Diversity at Work

A isha, a formidable presence at Mercy Mwongozo Hospital, understood the importance of fostering diversity and inclusivity in healthcare. She embarked on a mission to implement a thorough diversity training program to promote an inclusive environment where all clients and staff, regardless of their backgrounds, would feel valued and heard. She began her investigation by thoroughly analysing the hospital's existing practices and regulations. Aisha conducted surveys and focus groups with staff and clients to better understand their perspectives on diversity and inclusion. The discoveries from her initial research were genuinely enlightening and formed the foundation for creating her training program.

Aisha's diversity training program covered cultural competency, unconscious bias, and inclusive communication. She developed captivating workshops and seminars that provided valuable knowledge and fostered active engagement in thought-provoking discussions and introspection. These sessions were designed to question misunderstandings and promote a deeper understanding of clients' and colleagues' diverse needs and experiences.

Aisha's program placed great emphasis on scenario-based training. This training involved role-playing exercises where healthcare providers assumed clients' roles from diverse backgrounds. These exercises proved to be highly effective in fostering empathy and understanding among staff members, enabling them to understand better and address the unique challenges clients face from diverse cultural, religious, and socioeconomic backgrounds. In addition to training sessions, Aisha implemented a mentorship program that connected staff members from diverse backgrounds. This program fostered cross-cultural interactions and learning, fostering a more inclusive workplace atmosphere by breaking down barriers.

Aisha was also focused on attracting and retaining a diverse workforce. She worked closely with the hospital's human resources department to develop strategies that attracted candidates from various backgrounds and promoted a fair and unbiased recruitment process. This program not only brought a more comprehensive range of staff members but also introduced a variety of perspectives and backgrounds to the hospital, enhancing the quality of client care.

Aisha's diversity training program had a significant impact. Employees expressed a heightened understanding and value for cultural differences, leading to a more compassionate and individualised approach to client care. Clients experienced a noticeable improvement in how they were treated, resulting in increased satisfaction and overall happiness with the care they received.

Aisha's dedication extended beyond the training sessions as well. She established a diversity committee that consistently evaluated and improved the hospital's diversity and inclusivity practices. This committee served as a platform for ongoing dialogue and implementation, guaranteeing that diversity and inclusivity remained at the core of the hospital's mission.

As director of the diversity training program at Mercy Mwongozo Hospital, Aisha's personal growth and acceptance of diversity emerged. Her work demonstrated how fostering a more compassionate, wise, and inclusive hospital environment may be achieved via education and open discourse.

Her program has consistently motivated and guided, highlighting the vital importance of healthcare professionals in promoting diversity and inclusivity. Aisha's actions showcased a commitment to a healthcare system that values and appreciates the diverse range of human differences. Her work demonstrated that a diverse and inclusive healthcare environment enhances client care and enhances and fortifies the healthcare community as a whole.

Aisha's diversity training program profoundly impacted the culture of Mercy Mwongozo Hospital. The hospital staff started displaying a greater understanding and appreciation for cultural and individual differences, leading to improved and positive interactions between colleagues and clients. This transformation extended beyond the clinical sections and permeated every department, resulting in a friendlier and more inclusive environment across the hospital.

Aisha's remarkable achievements included creating treatment procedures that prioritised clients' needs and preferences, considering their ethnicity, religion, and personal choices. These protocols guided healthcare providers in delivering care that was not only medically sound but also culturally appropriate and respectful. Clients expressed a greater sense of being understood and valued, resulting in enhanced confidence and compliance with medical advice.

Aisha also emphasised the importance of language services at the hospital. She advocated for the inclusion of interpreters and the translation of essential healthcare documents into multiple languages. This project aimed to overcome language barriers to ensure seamless healthcare delivery and enhance client understanding and involvement in their treatment.

Aisha actively organised community engagement programs to foster diversity and inclusivity. These initiatives aimed to enhance connections with the numerous communities served by Mercy Mwongozo Hospital. By engaging in these outreach initiatives, the hospital gained valuable insights into the unique healthcare needs of its communities, strengthening its reputation as a reliable healthcare provider. The success of Aisha's program caught the interest of other healthcare organisations. She was sought after as a speaker, sharing her insights and perspectives at healthcare conferences and seminars, inspiring other organisations to embark on similar diversity and inclusion initiatives. Aisha's work started to significantly impact broader changes in healthcare practices, highlighting the importance of diversity and inclusion in delivering top-notch care.

Aisha's efforts have led to ongoing training and education programs. Understanding the ongoing nature of the journey towards inclusivity, she implemented yearly training sessions for all employees. This ensured that new hires were immersed in a culture of diversity and inclusion while providing existing staff with regular opportunities to enhance their skills and knowledge.

Aisha's experience managing the diversity training program at Mercy Mwongozo Hospital was genuinely remarkable. It was filled with unwavering commitment, transformative progress, and a strong focus on inclusivity. Her experience showcased the profound impact of a passionate individual in fostering an atmosphere that embraces diversity and incorporates inclusivity into every aspect of organisational culture.

Aisha's project has been a source of inspiration and influence, serving as a role model for healthcare organisations striving to create a more inclusive and compassionate healthcare environment. Her efforts demonstrated a solid commitment to a healthcare system that appreciates and embraces the diversity of its community, ensuring that every client and staff member is treated with utmost dignity and respect. Aisha's work showcased the power of proactive and conscientious efforts in creating a healthcare environment that is diverse, inclusive, and fair for everyone.

Aisha's endeavours fostered a more profound comprehension and embrace within the hospital, transcending conventional perspectives on healthcare delivery. Her diversity training program became a cornerstone of the hospital's character, shaping internal policy and how the institution interacted with the broader community. Aisha's program influenced client satisfaction scores, which saw a significant improvement. Clients from diverse backgrounds experienced greater comfort and comprehension, leading to enhanced care and better health results. This shift resulted from the staff's increased expertise in navigating cultural nuances and sensitivities in client care.

In addition, Aisha's dedication to promoting diversity also encompassed addressing health disparities within the community. She worked with local organisations to identify and address marginalised groups' unique health needs. This endeavour led to developing specialised health initiatives, including community health fairs, wellness programs, and health education sessions tailored to address these communities' specific challenges. Aisha initiated scholarship programs to support minority students in the healthcare field, demonstrating her dedication to fostering a diverse and inclusive healthcare workforce. These scholarships enabled students from varied backgrounds to pursue careers in healthcare, resulting in a more diverse healthcare workforce in the future.

Aisha's efforts to promote diversity and inclusion influenced the hospital's recruiting and retention strategies. The hospital gained a reputation for its inclusive approach, which drew on a broader pool of job candidates. Employee retention increased as they felt valued and respected, resulting in a more stable and experienced team. Aisha's work had an impact that reached beyond the boundaries of Mercy Mwongozo Hospital. She emerged as a highly regarded healthcare diversity and inclusion champion, influencing policies and practices at various hospitals and healthcare institutions. Other organisations adopted her methodology of diversity training, leading to significant reforms in the healthcare industry.

Aisha's efforts have significantly impacted the development of new client advocacy programs. These programs ensured that all clients' perspectives, especially those from marginalised communities, were considered and valued in healthcare decision-making. This endeavour reinforced the hospital's commitment to caring, prioritising clients and embracing diversity.

Aisha also coordinated global symposiums on healthcare diversity, uniting professionals from around the globe to exchange best practices and delve into ideas for promoting healthcare equity. These symposiums fostered a worldwide dialogue on diversity and inclusivity in healthcare, highlighting the universal significance of these principles. Aisha's remarkable journey leading the Mercy Mwongozo Hospital diversity training program is a powerful testament to the profound impact of embracing diversity and inclusivity in healthcare. Her journey showcased the profound effect of valuing and embracing diversity on creating a healthcare setting where everyone feels valued and supported.

Aisha's activities have continued to inspire and guide, serving as a shining example for healthcare facilities worldwide. Her work exemplified a commitment to a healthcare system that values and embraces diversity, ensuring that inclusivity is a fundamental aspect of delivering effective treatment. Aisha's endeavours illuminated the potential for hospitals to become havens of healing, respect, and harmony for everyone, showcasing the power of commitment, compassion, and proactive measures. Aisha's contributions to the healthcare community were far-reaching, particularly in developing a more inclusive health policy. She collaborated closely with legislators, offering insights and recommendations on how to make healthcare more accessible and egalitarian. Her efforts led to the implementation of laws that ensured healthcare services were accessible and responsive to the diverse needs of communities.

Aisha's training programs set a new standard for cultural competency training in healthcare settings. Her approach, which seamlessly integrated theoretical knowledge with practical, hands-on experiences, fostered a deep understanding and value for diversity among healthcare professionals. Furthermore, Aisha's actions sparked a change in client involvement tactics. The hospital staff was able to better connect with clients in their care due to their heightened awareness of each individual's diverse background. This transition increased client adherence to treatment programs, enhanced client-provider communication, and improved client outcomes.

Aisha assembled community advisory boards consisting of individuals from diverse ethnic backgrounds in her pursuit of fostering an inclusive environment. These boards played a crucial role in providing input and guidance on the hospital's healthcare services, ensuring that they were tailored to meet the needs of its diverse population.

Aisha's diversity program was so successful that it became integral to the hospital's onboarding procedure for new workers. Every new employee at Mercy Mwongozo Hospital undergoes comprehensive training on diversity and inclusion, ensuring that these values are deeply embedded in the hospital's culture. Furthermore, Aisha sparked several community health projects for neglected and marginalised populations. These projects had a dual purpose of providing healthcare services and educating communities about preventative healthcare, empowering them to take charge of their health.

Aisha's dedication to promoting diversity and inclusion at Mercy Mwongozo Hospital has made her a prominent figure in driving progressive change within the healthcare industry. Her experience highlighted the profound influence of fostering an atmosphere where individuals from diverse backgrounds are treated with kindness and courtesy.

Aisha's activities continued to inspire and guide, setting a benchmark for healthcare organisations around the globe. Her work showcased a solid commitment to a healthcare system that values diversity and aims to provide fair and inclusive care for everyone. Aisha's endeavours underscored the vital importance of healthcare professionals and institutions in driving societal transformation, stressing that embracing diversity and inclusivity is a moral obligation and essential for attaining excellence in healthcare.

As Aisha's diversity and inclusion program progressed, it started to influence not just client care but the overall atmosphere of the hospital as well. Due to the program's remarkable achievements, it has gained recognition as a crucial element of top-notch healthcare provision. This recognition led to a significant change in the hospital's culture, where diversity and inclusivity became integrated into the work of every department rather than being seen as separate initiatives.

The program's effectiveness was further showcased by the positive impact on health outcomes in communities where access to healthcare had previously been limited. Mercy Mwongozo Hospital successfully expanded its reach and served a more comprehensive range of the community by creating a more inclusive environment. This result was especially noticeable in locations where cultural differences had traditionally hampered effective healthcare delivery.

Aisha's dedication to inclusivity has led to the development of a comprehensive set of guidelines for client-centred care. These guidelines emphasised the importance of considering each client's unique cultural, language, and personal background when developing a care plan. These criteria ensured that client care was based on solid clinical principles, took into account cultural considerations, and was tailored to each individual. Aisha also developed a framework for consistently assessing and enhancing the diversity program. This system incorporates ongoing evaluations and modifications to ensure the training remains up-to-date and impactful. Staff and client feedback were crucial in this approach as it offered valuable real-world insights into the program's impact and areas for enhancement.

She significantly impacted other healthcare institutions through her dedication to diversity and inclusion, creating a network of hospitals and providers committed to enhancing healthcare equity. This network aimed to promote equal access to healthcare by organising conferences, fostering collaboration on projects, and facilitating the sharing of resources. In addition, Aisha's actions sparked academic interest, leading to research studies and publications on the impact of diversity and inclusivity in healthcare. The research provided empirical evidence supporting the effectiveness of Aisha's approaches, further validating her methodology.

Aisha's story of overseeing the diversity training program at Mercy Mwongozo Hospital is a remarkable testament to the transformative power of dedication, compassion, and ingenuity in healthcare. Her experience showcases the positive transformations that can occur when healthcare professionals and institutions dedicate themselves to understanding and meeting the diverse needs of their communities. Aisha's endeavours have consistently served as a source of inspiration and global impact, leading healthcare organisations worldwide to adopt a more varied and inclusive approach. Her efforts were a stark reminder of the need for healthcare professionals to foster a more equal and compassionate healthcare system. Aisha's endeavours demonstrated a commitment to establishing an inclusive healthcare setting that provided the highest quality of care to individuals from all walks of life.

CHAPTER 26

The Ethics of AI

As Aisha's diversity and inclusion program progressed, it started to influence not just client care but the overall atmosphere of the hospital as well. Due to the program's remarkable achievements, it has gained recognition as a crucial element of exceptional healthcare provision. This recognition led to a significant change in the hospital's culture, where diversity and inclusivity became integrated into the work of every department rather than being seen as separate initiatives.

The program's effectiveness was further highlighted by its positive impact on health outcomes in communities where access to healthcare had previously been limited. Mercy Mwongozo Hospital successfully expanded its reach and better served a more comprehensive range of the community by creating a more inclusive environment. This outcome was particularly evident in areas where cultural disparities had historically hindered efficient healthcare provision.

Aisha's dedication to inclusivity has led to the development of a comprehensive set of guidelines focused on client-centred care. These guidelines highlighted the significance of considering each client's cultural, language, and personal background when creating a care plan. These criteria ensured that client care was clinically sound and regarded as cultural sensitivity and personalised attention.

Aisha additionally developed a framework for consistently assessing and enhancing the diversity program. This system incorporates ongoing evaluations and modifications to ensure the training remains up-to-date and impactful. Staff and client feedback was crucial in this approach as it offered valuable real-world insights into the program's impact and areas for enhancement.

She significantly impacted other healthcare institutions through her dedication to diversity and inclusion, establishing a network of hospitals and providers committed to enhancing healthcare equity. This network was dedicated to the shared goal of promoting equal access to healthcare for everyone. They achieved this through organising conferences, collaborating on projects, and sharing resources.

In addition, Aisha's actions garnered academic interest, leading to research studies and publications on the impact of diversity and inclusivity in healthcare. The research provided solid evidence supporting the effectiveness of Aisha's approaches, further validating her methodology.

Aisha's story of overseeing the diversity training program at Mercy Mwongozo Hospital is a remarkable testament to the transformative power of dedication, compassion, and ingenuity in the healthcare industry. Her experience showcases the positive transformations that can occur when healthcare professionals and institutions dedicate themselves to understanding and meeting the diverse needs of their communities.

Aisha's endeavours continued to captivate and impact individuals globally, laying the groundwork for healthcare establishments worldwide to adopt a mindset of diversity and inclusiveness. Her endeavours served as a powerful reminder of the importance of healthcare professionals in cultivating a fair and empathetic healthcare system. Aisha's endeavours demonstrated a commitment to establishing an inclusive healthcare setting that provided the highest quality of care to individuals from all walks of life.

Aisha's diversity program at Mercy Mwongozo Hospital profoundly impacted how the community approached healthcare. Aisha expanded her program to address various factors influencing health outcomes, including poverty, education, and housing. This recognition of the interconnectedness of social determinants of health highlights her commitment to a comprehensive approach. She collaborated with community leaders and organisations to develop projects that tackled these more significant challenges, leading to a more holistic approach to health and well-being.

Her endeavours also led to the establishment of community health ambassador programs. Through these programs, people from diverse backgrounds underwent training to act as intermediaries between their communities and the hospital. These ambassadors played a vital role in educating their communities about health issues, promoting preventive healthcare, and making medical services more accessible.

In addition, Aisha's contributions became instrumental in shaping the hospital's policy on client rights and advocacy. Her ideas led to establishing regulations that guaranteed the protection of clients' rights, irrespective of their cultural or social background. The hospital's dedication to treating all clients fairly and respectfully was strengthened by its focus on client rights.

Aisha's diversity training program at Mercy Mwongozo Hospital gained recognition from international students and healthcare professionals. They arrived with a thirst for knowledge about the hospital's innovative approach to healthcare diversity and inclusion. This knowledge-sharing and experience enhanced the hospital's procedures and strengthened its reputation as a trailblazer in inclusive healthcare.

In addition, Aisha's dedication to diversity and inclusivity improved the hospital's marketing and communication efforts. The hospital has updated its public-facing assets, including its website and client information leaflets, to better represent the diverse communities it serves. This approach facilitated the cultivation of trust and enhanced the hospital's rapport with the community.

Aisha's experience leading the diversity training program at Mercy Mwongozo Hospital exemplified her exceptional leadership skills and commitment to fostering inclusivity. Her program showcased the power of dedication and a deep understanding of community needs in driving meaningful improvements in healthcare delivery and client outcomes.

Her work has consistently sparked inspiration and profoundly influenced others, serving as a paradigm for healthcare organisations across the globe. Aisha's endeavours demonstrated a commitment to establishing a healthcare setting where diversity is recognised and integrated into the essence of healthcare provision. Her work showcased the transformative power of inclusivity in healthcare, highlighting the importance of embracing diversity to deliver top-notch care and foster a more just and balanced society.

As Aisha's diversity and inclusion program expanded, it started to significantly impact both internal practices at Mercy Mwongozo Hospital and the overall approach to healthcare delivery. The program's impact permeated the organisation, fostering a more empathetic and culturally sensitive approach to client interactions. This transition was evident in the thoughtful attention clients received, which was customised to their unique cultural and personal requirements.

The growing body of research from collaborations between Mercy Mwongozo Hospital and academic institutions further enhanced the program's success. These studies provided evidence that diversity and inclusion training positively affect healthcare outcomes. The study's findings were published in renowned medical journals, contributing to the broader conversation about the importance of cultural competency in healthcare.

Aisha established client advisory councils with individuals from diverse backgrounds, demonstrating her commitment to fostering inclusivity. These councils offered a platform for individuals to share their concerns, insights, and recommendations, significantly influencing the hospital's policies and practices. This endeavour improved client care and empowered individuals to engage in healthcare actively.

In addition, Aisha's efforts started to influence how healthcare was taught and practised beyond the confines of Mercy Mwongozo Hospital. Other healthcare organisations started adopting similar diversity training programs, acknowledging the significance of these initiatives in enhancing client care and employee satisfaction. Aisha was often sought after to guide these programs, utilising her expertise and perspectives to support other organisations in crafting their diversity and inclusion strategies.

The success of the diversity training program resulted in its integration into the broader healthcare network. Aisha collaborated with various hospitals, clinics, and healthcare professionals to develop a unified strategy for promoting diversity and inclusivity in healthcare. This collaborative effort resulted in a more consistent and comprehensive approach to client care across various healthcare settings.

Aisha's contributions influenced the staff at Mercy Mwongozo Hospital. The diversity training program fostered a harmonious and cooperative workplace environment where every employee's worth and dignity were acknowledged, regardless of background. This positive work environment led to higher job satisfaction and reduced employee turnover rates, improving overall efficiency and effectiveness for the hospital.

Aisha also organised yearly discussions on diversity and inclusion at Mercy Mwongozo Hospital. These forums provided a platform for healthcare professionals, clients, community leaders, and diversity and inclusion specialists to discuss their experiences, challenges, and practical strategies. These gatherings became a hub for knowledge exchange and discussion, fostering a culture of ongoing development and advancement in healthcare diversity and inclusion.

Aisha's remarkable work at Mercy Mwongozo Hospital spearheading the diversity training program is a powerful testament to the profound impact of inclusive leadership in the healthcare sector. Her dedication showcased the sector's immense potential when it embraced diversity as a fundamental aspect of its operations.

Her work has consistently served as inspiration and guidance, setting a benchmark for healthcare organisations globally. Aisha's endeavours showcased a commitment to establishing a healthcare setting where everyone receives considerate, compassionate, and culturally sensitive care regardless of background. Her effort showcased the importance of acknowledging and embracing diversity in healthcare, highlighting that true excellence in healthcare delivery is achieved when inclusivity is prioritised in every action and decision.

After establishing a solid foundation, Aisha's diversity and inclusion program at Mercy Mwongozo Hospital has consistently grown to meet the evolving demographics and needs of the client population. She implemented regular program assessments to ensure their continued relevance and effectiveness in addressing current diversity-related healthcare concerns.

Aisha decided to incorporate virtual reality (VR) technology into diversity training. This technology provided immersive experiences that aided personnel in gaining a deeper understanding and empathy for clients from diverse backgrounds. VR scenarios encompassed a variety of situations that healthcare staff may not typically encounter, equipping them to handle various cultural exchanges and enhancing their proficiency in delivering culturally sensitive care.

Aisha also understood the importance of addressing disparities in health literacy. She developed educational materials and programs for clients with different literacy levels, ensuring that everyone comprehended their health conditions and the care they were receiving. This project had a profound effect on enhancing client engagement and compliance with treatment plans.

To foster inclusivity, Aisha expanded the scope of the diversity training to include various aspects of diversity, such as physical, cognitive, and neurological differences. She worked alongside experts to develop training modules that helped healthcare staff better comprehend and address the needs of impaired clients. This training was crucial in creating an inclusive atmosphere where every client received compassionate and professional care.

Aisha's work significantly influenced the hospital's community outreach programs. She launched initiatives to establish health clinics in marginalised communities, providing essential treatment and education. These clinics expanded healthcare access and served as a bridge between the hospital and the diverse communities, fostering trust and establishing lasting partnerships.

Aisha's diversity and inclusion program at Mercy Mwongozo Hospital significantly impacted healthcare policy at the state and national levels. Policymakers sought Aisha's expertise in integrating diversity and inclusivity into healthcare policy and practices on a broader scale. Her input played a crucial role in shaping policies addressing healthcare disparities and promoting equal access to healthcare.

Aisha's experience spearheading the diversity training program at Mercy Mwongozo Hospital is a testament to the transformative impact of dedicated leadership. Her project showcased the profound influence of embracing diversity and inclusion on the healthcare landscape, extending beyond just one institution.

Her work has consistently inspired and profoundly impacted healthcare providers and institutions globally. Aisha's actions demonstrated a solid commitment to a healthcare system that prioritises diversity and embraces inclusivity at every level. Her actions were a powerful reminder of the importance of acknowledging and appreciating diversity in healthcare, which is essential for delivering top-notch care and promoting a more equitable and healthier society.

Aisha's diversity program started to influence the broader healthcare community. Impressed by Mercy Mwongozo's achievements, hospitals and healthcare organisations contacted Aisha for assistance in creating comparable initiatives. This led to establishing a network of healthcare organisations committed to fostering diversity and inclusivity and sharing resources, challenges, and achievements.

Aisha's influence extended to medical and nursing institutions, where her strategies for inclusiveness were integrated into the instructional curriculum. This integration ensured that future healthcare professionals had the knowledge and understanding necessary to provide culturally sensitive care.

Aisha was recognised for her valuable contributions and invited to participate in national healthcare forums and task forces to address healthcare inequities. Her keen insights contributed to formulating comprehensive strategies and initiatives to foster a more equitable healthcare system. She advocated for policies that considered the clinical needs of different populations and the social and economic factors that impact their well-being.

In addition, Aisha spearheaded a range of community health initiatives focused on empowering clients to take an active role in their healthcare. Health education seminars, support groups, and community health fairs were organised to actively involve diverse community members and cater to their specific health needs.

Aisha's work significantly influenced the hospital's internal operations. Under her leadership, the hospital implemented policies and practices that promoted a diverse and inclusive environment for all staff. This approach led to a workforce with a broader range of perspectives, enhancing the hospital's capacity to understand and meet the unique needs of its clients.

Furthermore, Aisha's program started incorporating technology to expand its reach to a broader audience. She developed online training modules and virtual seminars to ensure that the principles of diversity and tolerance were effectively disseminated beyond the hospital's local boundaries.

Aisha's narrative of spearheading the diversity training initiative at Mercy Mwongozo Hospital is a compelling illustration of visionary leadership and a steadfast commitment to fostering inclusivity in the healthcare sector. Her narrative underscored the power of diligent effort and innovative thought in driving significant advancements in the provision and quality of healthcare.

Her work has been a source of inspiration and guidance, serving as a model for healthcare providers and institutions around the globe. Aisha's efforts showcased a solid commitment to a healthcare system that values and embraces diversity, fostering an inclusive environment. Her actions demonstrated a firm belief in embracing diversity and promoting tolerance to ensure top-notch care and create a fairer, more balanced society.

CHAPTER 27

Zara's Legislative Effort

Zara, known for her passionate support for healthcare reform at Mercy Mwongozo Hospital, was amid a significant parliamentary conflict. Her objective was to advocate for legislative reforms that would enhance access and quality of care for everyone. She quickly realised, though, that navigating the intricacies of healthcare policy would require determination, sharp intellect, and unwavering commitment.

She thoroughly analysed existing healthcare policies and their effects on the quality of client care. Zara identified critical areas for improvement, including ensuring clients can easily access care, making healthcare more affordable, and enhancing service quality. Armed with this knowledge, she gathered a group of healthcare experts, client advocates, and community leaders to rally behind her cause.

Zara's first move in tackling political hurdles was to arrange meetings with local and state legislators. She orchestrated gatherings and presentations to enlighten them about pressing healthcare issues and the necessity for change. She sought to highlight problems and offer practical solutions grounded in research.

Zara faced significant resistance in her campaign from numerous interest groups who were content with the status quo or had conflicting objectives. She tackled these challenges by fostering a culture of open discussion, seeking to understand different perspectives, and seeking areas of agreement. Her skill in effectively conveying ideas and building connections was crucial in achieving her goals.

Zara also acknowledged the impact of public sentiment on legislative decisions. She actively raised public awareness regarding pressing healthcare issues and proposed necessary enhancements. Engaging in community forums, reaching out on social media, and fostering collaborations with local media outlets were integral to these campaigns. Zara believed that through increasing public awareness, she could cultivate support from the community and compel policymakers to take action.

Zara's notable achievement was coordinating a healthcare symposium that united professionals, policymakers, and community members. The conference offered a platform for thoughtful conversations about healthcare issues and potential solutions. It facilitated the collaboration of numerous stakeholders and played a crucial role in developing a more cohesive and extensive reform program.

Zara faced numerous setbacks and challenges throughout her journey. On the other hand, her unwavering commitment and belief in the cause of healthcare reform fueled her perseverance. She was constantly refining her techniques, gaining insights from each event and perfecting her approach to lobbying and bargaining.

Zara's work at Mercy Mwongozo Hospital navigating legislative challenges in healthcare reform became a compelling tale of determination, guidance, and impact. Her experience showcased the crucial effect healthcare workers can have in advocating for legislative reforms that enhance client care and healthcare systems.

Zara's initiative continued to inspire and guide, showcasing how healthcare professionals can effectively engage in legislative advocacy. Her actions exemplified a commitment to ensuring a healthcare system that is fair, accessible, and of exceptional quality for everyone. Zara's work demonstrated that one could overcome political barriers through dedication and strategic efforts and significantly transform healthcare policy.

Zara's legislative initiatives gained momentum as she continued to attract support from a diverse range of sources. She understood that achieving meaningful healthcare reform necessitated a comprehensive approach involving changes in legislation, shifts in public attitudes, and advancements in healthcare practices.

She focused on cultivating connections with prominent healthcare stakeholders, including insurance companies, pharmaceutical firms, and healthcare providers. Zara facilitated discussions to link their passions with the objective of healthcare reform, emphasising the lasting advantages of a healthier society and a more streamlined healthcare system. Zara's insatiable curiosity drove her to explore groundbreaking healthcare approaches globally. She examined international healthcare systems that had successfully implemented reforms and extracted valuable insights that could be applied in her situation. Her advocacy was enhanced by this global perspective, offering concrete illustrations of effective healthcare policies and procedures.

Zara prioritised her efforts to advocate for the needs of marginalised communities. She aimed to guarantee that healthcare changes addressed the needs of individuals who often faced marginalisation in the healthcare system, including low-income families, the elderly, and people with chronic illnesses. Her approach emphasised the importance of having access to healthcare and ensuring that the care received is high-quality and consistent.

Zara gained recognition in the healthcare industry for her expertise in navigating the complex landscape of healthcare policy. Policymakers and healthcare leaders sought her advice and proposals. She started authoring articles and delivering speeches on healthcare reform, expanding her message and reaching a wider audience.

Zara's role also involved guiding and supporting aspiring healthcare professionals who were passionate about healthcare policy and activism. She understood the importance of cultivating a fresh wave of healthcare executives dedicated to reform and possessing the necessary skills to transform. Zara's story of overcoming legislative challenges in healthcare reform is a powerful testament to an individual's influence in policy and activism. Her journey showcased the impact of strategic and deliberate actions in transforming healthcare systems.

Zara's project has consistently motivated and supported healthcare professionals interested in participating in policy advocacy. Her initiatives showcased a solid commitment to creating a healthcare system that is accessible, affordable, and adaptable to the needs of all segments of society. Zara's dedication demonstrated that one can surmount political challenges and make meaningful contributions to healthcare reform through persistence, cooperation, and informed advocacy.

Zara's unwavering dedication to healthcare reform ignited significant discourse at the state and national levels. Her skill in effectively conveying intricate healthcare issues to lawmakers and the public was vital in her rise to prominence. She possesses a unique talent for simplifying complex medical terminology, effectively bringing the importance of healthcare reform beyond mere politics.

In her advocacy, Zara also delved into the financial aspects of healthcare. She worked with economists and healthcare financiers to develop models illustrating the potential cost savings of implementing comprehensive healthcare reform in the long run. These models demonstrated the potential impact of prioritising preventive care, improving access to medical services, and increasing investment in public health to reduce healthcare costs in the long run.

Zara orchestrated a sequence of community town halls to pursue her goal of catalysing transformation. At these gatherings, people could discuss their healthcare experiences with lawmakers, shedding light on the practical consequences of healthcare policy decisions. These poignant accounts from clients, carers, and healthcare professionals added a profound human element to the healthcare conversation, underscoring the urgent necessity for reform.

Zara understood the importance of the media in shaping public opinion and policy. She collaborated with journalists and media outlets, providing data, stories, and insights crucial to maintaining public awareness of healthcare reform. Her communication skills across various media outlets were critical to gaining public support for the planned reforms.

Zara's endeavours extended beyond altering existing policy; she was crucial in formulating innovative healthcare legislation. She collaborated with legal experts and lawmakers to develop legislation addressing critical healthcare system gaps. Her enthusiastic involvement ensured that the proposed bill was both practical and impactful.

Zara's work started gaining recognition and support from health organisations worldwide. Her work earned a new level of recognition on the global stage, opening up opportunities for international collaboration on health initiatives and policy. It also provided a worldwide platform for exchanging the successes and obstacles of Mercy Mwongozo Hospital's healthcare reform journey. Zara's efforts began to yield results. Several measures she advocated successfully improved healthcare access and quality in different communities. These achievements were a product of her astute approach, a knack for building alliances, and unwavering commitment to healthcare reform.

Zara remained committed to her profession as a healthcare practitioner throughout her journey. She worked closely with clients and healthcare providers, prioritising their perspectives and experiences to guide her advocacy efforts. This relationship helped her stay focused and reminded her of the ultimate purpose of her legislative efforts.

Zara's tireless dedication to overcoming legislative obstacles in healthcare reform is a testament to her unwavering determination, forward-thinking approach, and exceptional leadership skills. Her journey highlighted the significant impact that healthcare professionals could have in influencing policy and advocating for comprehensive improvements across the system.

Zara's campaign has consistently inspired and provided valuable guidance, establishing a solid foundation for impactful healthcare activism. Her initiatives showcased a strong commitment to establishing a healthcare system that is fair, enduring, and attuned to the needs of all individuals. Zara's work is a powerful reminder of the impact healthcare professionals can have on shaping policies that affect the health and well-being of entire communities. Their dedication, expertise, and intentional efforts make them influential agents of change.

Zara's advocacy career also connected her with technology professionals and data analysts to develop cutting-edge tools for healthcare policy analysis. These tools helped evaluate the potential effects of different healthcare policies, providing policymakers with evidence-based insights. This approach strengthened the argument for specific reforms and helped refine policy recommendations to achieve the highest effectiveness and efficiency.

Her passion for technology drove her to champion integrating digital health solutions into healthcare reform. Zara strongly supported the implementation of legislation that promoted telemedicine, electronic health records, and other digital tools to enhance healthcare access and quality, with a specific focus on rural and underserved areas. She recognised the potential of technology in bridging healthcare disparities and tirelessly advocated for incorporating this vision into legislative advancements.

Zara's initiatives further enhanced the focus on training and education in healthcare policy among medical professionals. She implemented programs and workshops to educate healthcare professionals about the significance of policy in shaping healthcare outcomes and how they can actively engage in advocacy. These programs were instrumental in cultivating a healthcare staff that is well-versed in policy matters and capable of driving meaningful reforms.

Zara's work had a significant influence on the academic community as well. Her activities and experiences served as case studies in public health and healthcare management courses, inspiring a new generation of healthcare professionals to engage in policy advocacy.

Zara also started contemplating the global impact of her work. She cultivated connections with healthcare advocates and officials across the globe, establishing a worldwide network committed to sharing best practices and gaining insights from diverse healthcare systems. This network evolved into a powerful global healthcare advocacy platform, advocating for reforms that transcend borders. Zara's story of overcoming legislative hurdles in healthcare reform is a testament to the strength of determination, knowledge, and teamwork in achieving transformative progress. Her experience demonstrated the power of effective advocacy and policy participation in enhancing healthcare systems.

Zara's project has inspired and guided healthcare professionals who are dedicated to making a difference through legislative influence and creating positive change. Her initiatives showcased a commitment to a healthcare system that is responsive, fair, forward-thinking, and flexible in addressing emerging challenges. Zara's work highlighted the significant impact healthcare professionals have on shaping policies that directly affect the health and well-being of communities globally.

As Zara's healthcare reform initiatives progressed, her focus shifted towards ensuring the sustainability of healthcare systems in the long run. She strongly supported measures that addressed immediate healthcare needs and guaranteed the long-term viability of healthcare services. This involved promoting increased investment in healthcare infrastructure, workforce development, and innovative healthcare delivery models capable of withstanding future challenges.

Zara's impact started to extend into the realm of public health. She dedicated herself to projects that emphasised the importance of preventive healthcare practices, recognising that taking proactive measures is crucial for reducing the burden on healthcare systems in the long run. She strongly supported initiatives that promoted community health programs, vaccination campaigns, and public awareness on crucial health matters.

Zara was highly intrigued by tackling the socioeconomic determinants of health through legislative reform. She understood the significant influence of housing, education, and socioeconomic status on health outcomes. Zara collaborated with lawmakers to formulate policies that tackled these broader factors, aiming to enhance health outcomes by addressing the fundamental roots of health inequalities.

Zara understood the significance of mental health in her commitment to comprehensive healthcare reform. She advocated for legislation that emphasised the importance of integrating mental health treatment into the healthcare system, highlighting the equal significance of psychological and physical well-being. Her efforts led to a greater understanding and reduced discrimination regarding mental health issues.

A series of significant victories characterised Zara's legislative advocacy progress, as she successfully pushed for the passage of policies she had passionately supported. These achievements were recognised not just within the hospital but also across the healthcare community. They were seen as pivotal in the journey towards a fairer and more efficient healthcare system.

Zara's journey also highlighted the importance of perseverance in activism. Despite numerous obstacles and setbacks, she remained committed to healthcare reform. Her unwavering determination served as a source of inspiration for countless individuals, demonstrating that meaningful transformation often requires continuous commitment and steadfast resolve.

Zara's journey through the complex landscape of healthcare reform serves as a beacon of inspiration and insight for those striving to enact positive change in the industry. Her journey showcases the profound impact an individual armed with knowledge, passion, and determination can make in reshaping healthcare policies.

Zara's campaign has consistently sparked inspiration and significantly influenced aspiring healthcare advocates and legislators.

Her initiatives showcased a solid commitment to a healthcare system that is not only accessible and affordable but also thorough, inclusive, and prepared to tackle future challenges. Zara's work demonstrated that through thoughtful advocacy, purposeful action, and working together, we could bring about meaningful changes that benefit communities across the globe.

CHAPTER 28

Cure the Healers

John, a committed healthcare professional at Mercy Mwongozo Hospital, spearheaded a revolutionary program centred on the welfare of healthcare workers. Initially a local initiative, his program swiftly garnered national recognition for its inventive approach and impressive results.

John's program focused on realising that healthcare professionals, often consumed by their dedication to others, occasionally neglected their health and well-being. He endeavoured to address this problem by creating a comprehensive support system to enhance healthcare workers' mental, emotional, and physical well-being.

As part of the program, workshops and seminars provided valuable insights into stress management, mindfulness, and self-care techniques; these seminars were designed to create an interactive and immersive learning experience for healthcare professionals, allowing them to develop self-care skills in a nurturing setting instead of traditional lectures.

John also implemented a peer support system within the hospital. Through shared experiences, this approach connected healthcare workers with colleagues who could provide empathy, understanding, and guidance. The peer support system proved invaluable for healthcare workers, offering a secure space to discuss concerns and seek assistance.

One of the standout aspects of John's program was its incorporation of unconventional wellness techniques. Yoga, meditation, and art therapy sessions were provided, offering healthcare staff a range of options to discover what suited their stress-relief needs.

As the program progressed, John implemented feedback systems to enhance and adjust it continuously. He actively sought participant feedback to ensure that the program stayed up-to-date and effective in addressing the constantly evolving challenges that healthcare professionals face.

"Healing the Healers" at Mercy Mwongozo Hospital received widespread recognition, was published in esteemed medical journals, and was presented at prestigious healthcare conferences. John was requested to discuss the program's structure, its outcomes, and its positive improvements in the hospital's workplace.

In addition, hospitals across the country became aware of the program and expressed interest in duplicating it. John collaborated with various healthcare organisations to create and execute the program in different environments, considering a range of organisational cultures and requirements.

The widespread recognition of John's program shed light on a crucial aspect of healthcare that had previously been overlooked: healthcare professionals' physical and mental health. It started a conversation about the significance of caring for those who dedicate themselves to caring for others. John's experience with the program evolved into a tale of empathy and transformative growth. His endeavour showcased the potential benefits of prioritising the well-being of healthcare personnel, enhancing their own lives, and elevating the standard of care provided to clients.

He has continued to be a source of inspiration and guidance, serving as a nationwide role model for healthcare facilities. John's actions demonstrated a solid commitment to fostering a healthcare environment that values the well-being of both carers and clients. His work showed that prioritising healthcare practitioners' well-being could significantly enhance healthcare quality and effectiveness.

John started collaborating with mental health professionals to improve the program as his reputation grew. He integrated evidence-based psychological tactics, including cognitive-behavioural techniques, into the sessions, enhancing their efficacy in stress management and burnout prevention among healthcare workers.

John also understood the importance of leadership support in the program's success. He worked closely with hospital administration to seamlessly incorporate the program into the institution's operating procedures. The program received strong support from higher-ups, ensuring that participation was encouraged and seen as a crucial part of the hospital's dedication to its staff.

Sophistic tracking methods were implemented to monitor the program's impact. John and his team employed surveys and performance measures to evaluate employee well-being and job satisfaction improvements. The impressive results of these evaluations provided compelling evidence of the program's value, leading to its implementation in more hospitals.

It started providing private counselling services alongside organised courses and support from fellow members. This provided healthcare practitioners with a confidential space to seek assistance for personal and professional matters. Counselling services became an essential program component, offering individuals personalised support.

The program's national recognition opened up opportunities for research collaborations. John worked closely with academic institutions to study the program's effect on healthcare outcomes. The research findings highlighted the connection between the well-being of healthcare workers and the quality of client care, adding a new perspective to the ongoing discussion on healthcare efficiency and effectiveness.

John's efforts also piqued interest in policy circles. Deliberations on integrating similar programs into national healthcare plans commenced. Policymakers met with John to explore incorporating healthcare workers' well-being into broader healthcare reform initiatives.

John's story of involvement is a compelling testament to the vital importance of addressing healthcare professionals' needs for the healthcare system's overall well-being. His journey was a powerful reminder of the human element in healthcare, highlighting the significance of supporting carers in building strong and effective healthcare systems.

They continued to inspire and influence, setting a standard for healthcare organisations to prioritise the health and well-being of their employees. John's actions demonstrated a solid commitment to nurturing a healthcare culture that recognises the importance of the well-being of those involved in providing care as an integral part of the healthcare mission. His work showcased the belief that establishing a nurturing and positive work atmosphere for healthcare professionals is vital for delivering top-notch client care and maintaining a sustainable healthcare system.

John's program expanded into a comprehensive health initiative beyond the confines of Mercy Mwongozo Hospital. The program's success led to partnerships with universities, becoming part of the healthcare curriculum, and teaching upcoming healthcare professionals about the importance of self-care and mental well-being.

Understanding the link between physical and mental well-being, John decided to enhance the program by including regular health assessments, exercise routines, and nutritional guidance for healthcare professionals. He collaborated with fitness professionals and dietitians to create personalised wellness regimens, emphasising the importance of physical health in the program.

The program also began to explore the concept of work-life balance, acknowledging that healthcare professionals often face challenges in maintaining clear boundaries between personal and professional lives. John conducted training sessions on time management, setting healthy boundaries, and recognising the importance of taking breaks. These sessions helped healthcare staff improve their task management skills while prioritising their well-being.

One of the program's innovative aspects was incorporating technology to offer support. John created a digital platform that provided healthcare staff with stress management information, tips, and tools around the clock. This network also facilitated healthcare professionals' engagement and sharing of their experiences and coping strategies through a confidential peer-to-peer support system.

John's dedication to enhancing the welfare of healthcare staff started to influence hospital policies regarding work hours, shift rotations, and breaks. Hospitals that implemented the program experienced a decrease in worker burnout and absenteeism, along with an enhancement in job satisfaction and productivity.

The program's success led to its recognition as a model for healthcare worker wellness. John was invited to national and international healthcare forums to discuss the program and its impact, which motivated other healthcare facilities to adopt similar approaches.

In addition, John's diligent work made a noticeable difference in the quality of client care. Healthcare staff experienced an improvement in client care as they developed a deeper understanding of their well-being. Healthcare staff demonstrated heightened presence, empathy, and effectiveness, improving client satisfaction and outcomes.

The program's emphasis on mental health also contributed to reducing the stigma surrounding mental health issues in the healthcare sector. "Healing the Healers promoted the importance of healthcare staff reaching out for help when needed, fostering a supportive and empathetic workplace environment.

Furthermore, John's project ignited research on the influence of healthcare workers' well-being on the broader healthcare system. The research findings provided valuable insights into how healthcare worker wellness programs can be optimised for maximum impact.

The story of John's work took on a profound and inspiring narrative of innovation, empathy, and personal growth. His dedication showcased the potential for a healthcare system that values the health and well-being of its workers, leading to increased compassion, efficiency, and effectiveness.

Has consistently motivated and guided healthcare organisations globally. John's endeavours demonstrated a commitment to fostering a healthcare environment where the well-being of healthcare professionals is recognised as crucial to the overall mission of healthcare. His research showed the importance of prioritising the well-being of carers to ensure the long-term viability and effectiveness of healthcare systems worldwide.

John's program started to make a difference for healthcare personnel and the families and communities they served. Understanding the importance of healthcare workers' mental and emotional health in their job performance, the program started incorporating events and activities that focus on family and personal well-being. These events focused on establishing the support systems surrounding healthcare personnel, acknowledging the significance of family and community in an individual's holistic well-being.

The program has also started to gain attention from health insurance companies. Appreciating the enduring advantages of such wellness initiatives, numerous insurers started offering support and financial resources, seeing it as a forward-thinking investment in the well-being of healthcare professionals. This support helped to broaden the program's reach and resources, enabling John to provide a broader range of comprehensive wellness options.

In addition, John's approach started to break down established healthcare hierarchies. "Healing the Healers" fostered a strong sense of camaraderie and solidarity among hospital workers by providing a platform for all staff members, regardless of their roles, to gather and offer each other valuable support. This modification improved coworker relationships and cultivated a more collaborative and empathetic work environment.

As the program's reputation grew, John created a training and certification program for other organisations looking to launch similar initiatives. This training ensured that core principles and methodologies were upheld while accommodating diverse organisational cultures and requirements.

John also started considering the program's long-term sustainability. He dedicated himself to developing a long-term model that could function and adapt independently. This involved training a dedicated group to oversee and manage the program, guaranteeing its lasting effectiveness and influence.

Furthermore, a comprehensive report was compiled, highlighting the program's achievements and the positive feedback received from participants. This report, which showcased the profound changes experienced by the participants, proved to be a compelling resource in advocating for the importance of healthcare worker well-being in various healthcare environments.

John's work took on a captivating narrative, showcasing the transformative power of supporting those who dedicate themselves to caring for others within the healthcare system. His program highlighted the significance of emphasising healthcare workers' emotional and physical well-being in client care and the community's overall health.

"Healing the Healers" has consistently served as a source of inspiration and guidance, setting a standard for healthcare institutions globally. John's efforts showcased a solid commitment to fostering a healthcare culture that values and supports carers. His work was a powerful reminder of the interconnectedness between the health of healthcare personnel, the clients they care for, and the wider community. With "Healing the Healers," John developed a healthcare approach that is sustainable, compassionate, and encompasses the whole person.

As time passed, it focused on providing immediate relief from stress and ensuring healthcare personnel's long-term satisfaction and growth. John included career coaching and professional development sessions in the program. These programs supported healthcare professionals in defining career goals, acquiring new skills, and exploring innovative avenues for professional advancement.

John also acknowledged the healthcare staff's hard work and dedication. He created an annual recognition ceremony at Mercy Mwongozo Hospital to celebrate workers' dedication to client care, self-care, and health. This event boosted morale and highlighted the program's fundamental principles of gratitude and assistance.

In addition, John's initiative started to influence policy at a more elevated level. Hospitals and healthcare organisations initiated policy reforms that prioritised the well-being of their employees. Changes included implementing more flexible scheduling, increasing staff-to-client ratios, and incorporating wellness spaces within healthcare facilities. The influence was also evident in the reduction of mental health stigma within the healthcare profession. The program's open discussions and focus on mental well-being led to a significant change in how healthcare personnel viewed and talked about mental health. This openness allowed more healthcare workers to seek help and support when necessary.

Furthermore, John collaborated with esteemed scholars to analyse the program's impact on healthcare outcomes over an extended period. A correlation was discovered between the well-being of healthcare professionals and the satisfaction, safety, and quality of care experienced by clients. These findings provide valuable insights into the potential benefits of optimising the design of such programs to benefit both healthcare personnel and clients.

The program's achievements and influence on the lives of healthcare workers were extensively publicised, serving as a source of motivation for other organisations. John's work started gaining recognition at healthcare conferences, webinars, and magazines, spreading the message of carer well-being to a broader audience.

John's story exemplifies the significance of empathy, support, and community in the healthcare industry. His program showcased the potential for a more empathetic, streamlined, and prosperous healthcare system by focusing on the needs of healthcare workers. Has consistently motivated and guided, setting a precedent for healthcare organisations globally. John's efforts demonstrated a commitment to fostering a healthcare culture that values and acknowledges the personal needs of carers. His work emphasised the importance of prioritising the health and well-being of healthcare workers for the long-term sustainability and excellence of service. With "Healing the Healers," John advocated for a healthcare model that places the well-being of people at its core, particularly the healthcare practitioners themselves.

CHAPTER 29

Innovations in Geriatrics

Grace, a compassionate and progressive Mercy Mwongozo Hospital nurse, redirected her focus and expertise towards enhancing care for the elderly. She understood the importance of giving proper medical care and being well-informed about the specific challenges faced by the elderly population. Her innovative aged-care practices started to establish new standards in senior healthcare.

Grace developed a comprehensive care plan that extended beyond conventional medical treatments upon gaining insight into the distinct requirements of elderly individuals. This approach involved thorough evaluations that considered the older clients' overall well-being, including their physical health and mental, emotional, and social aspects.

Grace's contribution to the field of memory care therapies was genuinely groundbreaking. Music therapy, reminiscence therapy, and art therapy were all integrated into the care plans. These therapies not only brought pleasure to the clients but also helped maintain cognitive functioning and offered emotional support, enhancing the quality of life for individuals with dementia and Alzheimer's.

Grace also tried to enhance the geriatric ward's physical environment to better accommodate senior clients. She advocated revamping client rooms and common areas to ensure they were secure, cosy, and conducive to healing. Enhancements were made to the lighting, flooring, and accessibility features, along with inviting communal areas for clients to engage in socialising and various activities.

Grace made significant advancements in medication management. She worked alongside chemists to create improved methods for managing medication, recognising the challenges and dangers of polypharmacy in older adults. This approach significantly enhanced client safety by reducing prescription errors and adverse drug reactions.

Grace acknowledged the importance of supporting carers in senior care in addition to these advancements. She facilitated training workshops for family members and carers, equipping them with the necessary skills and knowledge to provide adequate care at home. This course delved into chronic illness management, nutrition, and emergency response.

Grace's approach to geriatric care also highlighted the importance of treating seniors with dignity and respect. She educated her team on effectively interacting with older individuals, ensuring their dignity, and promoting their autonomy in making decisions regarding their care.

Grace's groundbreaking advancements in geriatric care had a profound influence. Clients in the geriatric ward experienced improved health outcomes, increased levels of happiness, and an enhanced overall quality of life. The new strategy brought greater satisfaction to the personnel, enabling them to provide more thorough and compassionate treatment.

Other healthcare organisations started to pay attention to Grace's work in geriatric advancements. She has been invited to speak at conferences and seminars, where she has generously shared her expertise and insights with other healthcare professionals. Her methods quickly gained recognition and were adopted by numerous hospitals and care facilities, revolutionising the approach to geriatric care nationwide.

Grace's work in geriatric care at Mercy Mwongozo Hospital is a testament to her compassion, creativity, and unwavering commitment to improving the lives of the elderly. Her journey showcased the profound impact that intelligent and comprehensive approaches to healthcare for older people can make.

Grace's initiative inspired and guided others, setting a new benchmark for senior care. Her efforts showcased a commitment to a healthcare system that prioritises the well-being and needs of older people, ensuring they receive the dignity, respect, and care they deserve. Her work was a powerful testament to the importance of continually innovating and adapting healthcare practices to meet clients' evolving needs, particularly those in delicate stages of life.

Grace's understanding of geriatric care deepened as she gained more knowledge about the unique requirements of elderly individuals. She developed personalised exercise programs after recognising the significance of mobility and physical activity in preserving health and autonomy. These programs, led by physical therapists, were designed to enhance strength, balance, and flexibility, reducing fall risk and improving overall bodily function.

Grace also emphasised the significance of nutrition, a crucial aspect of geriatric care that needs to be considered. She collaborated with dietitians to create nutrition plans customised for the unique dietary requirements of older adults, guaranteeing that meals were both nourishing and enjoyable to eat. This comprehensive approach to nutrition helped address common challenges like malnutrition and weight loss in older individuals.

Grace seamlessly integrated technology into her care methods to deliver comprehensive care. She employed telemedicine to enhance healthcare accessibility for older individuals who faced challenges in regularly visiting the hospital. Telehealth sessions have been utilised for routine check-ups, consultations, and even specific treatment sessions, enhancing the accessibility and convenience of healthcare for senior individuals.

Grace also highlighted the importance of mental health treatment in her approach to geriatric care. She incorporated mental health evaluations and counselling options to tackle issues like depression, anxiety, and isolation, which are prevalent among older individuals. Focusing on mental health was crucial in providing a well-rounded approach to senior care.

Grace initiated various initiatives in the geriatric ward to foster a sense of community, recognising the significance of social interaction. She organised group activities and social events to promote client engagement and combat feelings of isolation and loneliness. These activities not only boosted the clients' social well-being but also had a positive impact on their overall health.

As Grace's program gained popularity, she passionately advocated for national policy reforms in geriatric care. She worked closely with healthcare policymakers to highlight the importance of increased resources, improved training, and elevated standards of care for older people. Her advocacy highlighted the issues older people face in healthcare legislation.

The improved quality of life experienced by the clients under Grace's care is a testament to the success of her groundbreaking advancements in geriatric care. Relatives of elderly clients often conveyed their gratitude for the thorough and compassionate care their loved ones received, underscoring the importance of Grace's diligent work.

Grace's groundbreaking work in senior care at Mercy Mwongozo Hospital is an inspiring testament to the transformative power of innovative and compassionate healthcare for elderly clients. Her study highlighted the importance of customising healthcare approaches to meet clients' specific needs at different stages of life.

Grace's initiatives continued to inspire and guide, setting a compassionate and successful standard for senior care. Her endeavours demonstrated a commitment to a healthcare system that values and cares for older people with dignity and consideration. Her work was a powerful testament to the importance of continuous innovation and dedication to enhancing healthcare for clients of all ages.

Grace's dedication to geriatric care prompted her to explore incorporating advanced technologies and digital tools to enhance aged care. She was a pioneer in utilising wearable sensors to track vital signs and identify potential health risks at an early stage. These devices allowed for ongoing monitoring of elderly clients, providing valuable data that could be used to adjust treatment strategies promptly.

Grace developed VR experiences specifically for older clients, understanding the power of virtual reality (VR) to enhance cognitive stimulation. These experiences aimed to stimulate clients mentally and emotionally, offering a break from the hospital environment and stimulating their memory and senses.

Grace's program also started to focus on end-of-life care, guaranteeing that elderly clients received caring and dignified treatment during their last days. She worked diligently to foster a warm and inclusive atmosphere for clients and their loved ones, incorporating palliative care principles and offering bereavement counselling and support services.

Grace collaborated with architects and designers to reimagine the architecture of elderly care facilities. She imagined secure, functional, aesthetically pleasing, and cosy rooms. The remodelled facilities were designed to enhance the quality of life for senior individuals by incorporating features such as natural lighting, easy navigation, and spaces that encourage social interaction.

Grace highlighted the significance of spiritual well-being in providing comprehensive care. She ensured clients had access to spiritual care services, respecting and accommodating the diverse religious and spiritual needs of older people under her care.

Grace established partnerships with nearby universities and research institutions as her program grew. These collaborations have fostered research in ageing and senior care, leading to a deeper understanding of optimal practices in aged care. The research findings were utilised to consistently enhance and innovate the care provided at Mercy Mwongozo Hospital.

The effectiveness of Grace's senior care program caught the attention of healthcare officials and leaders. Her approach to care was seen as a blueprint for transforming aged care nationwide. Grace was often invited to speak at national healthcare conferences and policy forums, where she shared her expertise and passionately advocated for increased emphasis and funding on aged care.

Grace's program also profoundly influenced geriatric care workers. Due to the noticeable improvements in client health and satisfaction, they expressed greater fulfilment and motivation. The program fostered a culture of empathy and creativity, drawing in healthcare professionals passionate about delivering quality care to older people.

Grace's work in senior innovations at Mercy Mwongozo Hospital is a remarkable tale of compassion, ingenuity, and unwavering commitment to the well-being of the elderly. Her journey demonstrated the profound impact of compassionate, client-focused care on improving the well-being of elderly individuals.

Grace's endeavours continued to inspire and guide, setting an example for empathetic and progressive geriatric care. Her efforts exemplified a commitment to a healthcare system that offers the compassion, consideration, and comprehensive care that older clients require. Her work was a powerful reminder of the importance of adapting healthcare methods to meet the evolving needs of an ageing population, ensuring their final stages are as comfortable and fulfilling as possible.

Grace's innovative approach to geriatric care started to impact the broader healthcare community, leading to a reconsideration of how elderly care was provided in various settings. Her achievement at Mercy Mwongozo Hospital established a new standard for other hospitals, showcasing the advantages of comprehensive and technologically advanced care for the elderly.

Grace developed outreach programs that fostered connections between older people and local volunteers and organisations, highlighting the importance of community engagement in elderly care. These programs enabled social connections and community involvement among older people, reducing feelings of isolation and cultivating a sense of belonging and purpose.

Grace's dedication to geriatric care extended to providing education and support for carers. She facilitated workshops and support groups for family members of elderly clients, supplying them with the necessary knowledge and tools to care for their loved ones effectively. These sessions delved into topics such as effectively managing chronic illnesses, gaining a deeper understanding of ageing, and navigating the complexities of caregiving challenges.

Grace highlighted the importance of regular mental health exams for older people in her pursuit of comprehensive care. She understood that within this particular group, mental health disorders often went unnoticed and unaddressed. She ensured that older clients received mental health services in a timely and sufficient manner by incorporating mental health screenings into their regular care.

Grace's work in senior care also started to impact policy at a higher level. Her innovative ideas and the remarkable impact of her Mercy Mwongozo Hospital program have influenced policy discussions on aged care. As a result, more comprehensive and age-friendly healthcare legislation has been developed.

The program's achievements were reflected in the improved quality of life experienced by the elderly clients and their families, going beyond mere figures and data. Clients under Grace's care often experienced notable enhancements in their physical and mental well-being, prompting their families to express sincere gratitude for their compassionate and thorough care.

Grace's dedication to transforming geriatric care at Mercy Mwongozo Hospital is a powerful testament to the potential of innovative thinking, compassion, and unwavering resolve to bring about meaningful change in the healthcare field. Her research highlighted the significance of a healthcare system that addresses the medical needs of older adults and supports their overall welfare.

Grace's initiatives continued to inspire and guide, setting new standards for aged care. Her efforts showcased a commitment to a healthcare system that values and honours the unique needs of older people, providing them with the utmost dignity and comprehensive care they merit. Her work highlighted the importance of continuous innovation and compassionate care in addressing the evolving needs of an ageing population and ensuring that their later years are filled with the utmost care and respect.

Grace's contributions to geriatric care started to shape society's perspective on ageing and the care of older people. She advocated for a shift in perspective, where ageing is seen as a valuable phase of life that should be honoured and provided with high-quality care rather than being seen as a decline. Her endeavours sparked a greater understanding among the public regarding the needs and potential of the ageing population.

Grace implemented intergenerational programs that united the younger and older generations, showcasing her commitment to enhancing elderly care. These programs fostered a mutual learning and understanding culture, challenging preconceived notions based on age. The older generation imparted wisdom and life lessons to the younger ones, who, in turn, found joy and a sense of purpose in interacting with their elders.

Grace also emphasised the importance of maintaining consistent care for elderly clients transitioning from the hospital to home care. She developed a thorough discharge planning process that included clients, their families, and a diverse team of healthcare providers. This process ensured that the elderly received consistent and coordinated care, decreasing hospital readmission rates and improving overall health outcomes.

In addition, Grace's geriatric care programs started to influence the design of medical equipment and gadgets. She collaborated with manufacturers to develop medical equipment tailored to the needs and abilities of older people, ensuring it was easy to use. This equipment was designed to enhance the healthcare experiences of senior individuals, guaranteeing ease of use and reducing any feelings of intimidation.

Grace's work dramatically influences the training and development of healthcare professionals specialising in geriatric care. She crafted a curriculum highlighting a compassionate and comprehensive approach to senior care, instructing healthcare professionals to consider more than just clinical symptoms and understand the broader context of each elderly client's life.

Grace's efforts also led to developing community-based healthcare models focused on proactive and preventive care for older people. These methods aimed to promote the well-being and engagement of older individuals within their communities to minimise the need for hospitalisation.

The story of Grace's endeavours at Mercy Mwongozo Hospital to revolutionise senior care became a shining example of ingenuity and empathetic treatment. Her experience underscored the importance of a deep understanding of the unique needs of older people, along with innovative approaches and technologies, in improving their quality of life.

Grace's innovative ideas continued to captivate and shape, ushering in a fresh era of senior care. Her actions showcased a commitment to a healthcare system that values the well-being of older people, treating them with dignity, courtesy, and a deep understanding of their unique requirements. Her work highlighted the importance of providing comprehensive, compassionate, and top-notch care to older people, ensuring they can enjoy their later years with good health, dignity, and happiness.

CHAPTER 30

Overcoming Burnout

Noah, a nurse at Mercy Mwongozo Hospital, became more aware of the escalating burnout among his nursing colleagues. After witnessing the toll that long hours, high stress, and emotional strain were taking on nurses, he decided to take action. Noah's dedication to advocating for improvements in nursing work settings has played a crucial role in raising awareness about this critical issue.

To uncover the underlying causes of burnout, he embarked on a comprehensive research endeavour, administering thorough surveys and conducting in-depth interviews with the nursing staff. The findings were surprising, revealing concerns such as understaffing, limited support, and inadequate breaks. With this knowledge, Noah initiated a crusade to increase understanding of nurse burnout and its impact on healthcare providers and client care quality.

Noah approached burnout from a diverse perspective. He advocated for higher staffing ratios, asserting that overworked nurses may be unable to provide adequate client care. He tirelessly dedicated himself to conveying this message to hospital executives and healthcare officials, stressing the significance of improving nurse staffing ratios and the safety and quality of client care.

Aside from staffing concerns, Noah expressed worry regarding the mental well-being of nurses. He strongly supported the implementation of regular mental health check-ins and support programs within the facility. His goal was to establish a work environment that fostered support for nurses and provided them with the necessary resources to cope with the challenges of their profession.

Noah also emphasised the importance of rest and rehabilitation for nurses. He advocated for increased flexibility in scheduling and mandatory breaks between shifts. He recognised the importance of nurses, just like any other individuals, having sufficient time to rejuvenate. He understood that working extended shifts without adequate breaks could harm their overall well-being and ability to provide effective client care.

Noah initiated a peer mentorship program upon recognising the significance of communal and peer assistance. Experienced nurses were paired with new employees to offer guidance, assistance, and a sympathetic ear. This program not only helped new nurses navigate the challenges of the job but also fostered a sense of camaraderie and mutual support among the nursing staff.

As Mercy Mwongozo Hospital began implementing some of Noah's improvements, the true impact of his efforts became evident. The hospital observed a rise in nurse morale, a decline in turnover rates, and a Mwongozo enhancement in the quality of client care.

Noah's accomplishments were acknowledged through invitations to speak at various healthcare forums and nursing conferences. His message resonated with healthcare professionals nationwide, sparking discussions on the systemic changes needed in nurse work environments nationwide.

Noah's efforts at Mercy Mwongozo Hospital to address burnout in the nursing profession became a tale of perseverance, advocacy, and hope. His journey showcased the profound influence of handling personnel matters on the healthcare system.

Noah's project has continued inspiring and guiding, showcasing how healthcare institutions can support and develop their nursing staff. His actions demonstrated a commitment to a healthcare system that values its employees' welfare as highly as its clients' treatment. Noah's work highlighted the importance of creating nurturing and sustainable work environments for nurses, guaranteeing they receive the necessary resources and support to excel in their crucial roles.

Noah's campaign against nurse burnout started to inspire change beyond the walls of Mercy Mwongozo Hospital. His efforts caught the interest of healthcare managers and lawmakers at both state and national levels, sparking more comprehensive discussions about the working conditions of nurses in different healthcare settings.

He began collaborating with national nursing organisations to advocate for policy enhancements. These included suggestions for the most extended duration of shifts, mandatory intervals between shifts, and policies promoting mental health resources for nurses. Noah's passionate advocacy highlighted the significance of these reforms for nurses and upholding exceptional standards of client care.

Noah also initiated a series of workshops and seminars for nurses, focusing on stress management and resilience-building. These workshops equipped nurses with practical tools and methods to handle the demanding nature of their profession effectively. The discussion covered various subjects, including mindfulness, effective communication, and healthy work-life balance strategies.

Noah also highlighted the importance of leadership training for nursing workers. He was convinced that equipping nurses with strong leadership skills would enable them to advocate for themselves and their colleagues effectively. This training also aimed to cultivate future nursing leaders who could carry on the mission of supporting improved working conditions.

Noah's work also initiated a research project to explore the impact of nurse burnout on client care. This study offered vital insights that Noah utilised to bolster his argument for systemic enhancements. The research uncovered a clear link between the well-being of nurses and the outcomes for clients, underscoring the need for improvements in nurse working conditions.

Noah launched a public awareness campaign upon recognising the importance of garnering public backing. He utilised a range of media platforms to highlight the challenges nurses face and their crucial contributions to the healthcare field. This campaign sparked public awareness and garnered support from many community groups, who joined Noah in advocating for enhanced working conditions for nurses.

The narrative of Noah's endeavours to address nursing burnout at Mercy Mwongozo Hospital and beyond unfolded as a captivating chronicle of advocacy, perseverance, and profound transformation. His journey highlighted the nurses' crucial role in the healthcare system and the significance of prioritising their well-being to enhance client care.

Noah's activities served as a source of inspiration and influence for others, setting a standard for addressing nursing burnout in healthcare systems across the globe. His initiatives showcased a solid commitment to fostering a healthcare environment that recognises and appreciates the contributions of nursing staff. Noah's work demonstrated the importance of supporting those who provide care to uphold a high-quality, efficient, and empathetic healthcare system.

Noah's endeavours transformed the atmosphere at Mercy Mwongozo Hospital and beyond. His endeavours led to increasing recognition of the importance of prioritising nurses' well-being as a crucial factor in the overall effectiveness of healthcare systems. The reforms he championed went beyond reducing stress and preventing burnout. They aimed to create an atmosphere where nurses could flourish and provide their clients with the highest level of care.

Noah developed a comprehensive wellness program for nurses in his ongoing endeavours. Regular health evaluations, fitness sessions tailored to the needs of healthcare workers, and nutritional counselling were all included in this program. Noah's aim in addressing physical health was to provide nurses with increased energy and resilience to meet the demands of their vocation.

Noah also sparked a series of hospital-wide collaborative discussions. These forums provided a platform for nurses to discuss their concerns, share their experiences, and collaborate on solutions to common challenges. By promoting open communication and collaboration, these forums fostered a stronger sense of community and support among the nursing staff.

Noah developed a 'Nurse of the Month' initiative after recognising the significance of acknowledgement and commendation in enhancing morale. This program highlighted nurses' diligent efforts and unwavering commitment, acknowledging the recognition they rightfully deserved. It improved morale and nurtured a high standards and empathy culture among the nursing team.

Noah's work had a profound effect on the clients as well. By fostering an environment of support and reducing stress levels, nurses enhanced client interactions, increasing client satisfaction and improved outcomes. The nursing staff's positive adjustments had a ripple effect, improving the hospital's overall care environment.

Noah's endeavours also significantly influenced nursing education. He collaborated with nursing schools to incorporate self-care, stress management, and resilience courses into the nursing curriculum.

This training ensured that new nurses were well-equipped to handle the profession's challenges and had established protocols to prioritise their well-being.

Noah's work in addressing nurse burnout was also acknowledged nationally. He was invited to participate in national healthcare policy debates, where he advocated for systemic changes to improve nurses' working conditions nationwide. His ideas and suggestions started to significantly impact national healthcare policies, particularly regarding the well-being of healthcare professionals.

Noah's efforts at Mercy Mwongozo Hospital to address nursing burnout unfolded as a compelling narrative of transformation, empowerment, and advocacy. His story showcased the significant impact of offering support to healthcare professionals on the overall healthcare system.

Noah's initiatives have consistently inspired and made a significant impact on individuals across the globe, serving as a role model for healthcare organisations worldwide. His actions demonstrated a solid commitment to fostering a healthcare culture that recognises nurses' vital roles and prioritises their well-being. Noah's work showcased the idea that when healthcare systems prioritise the well-being and support of nurses, it can lead to improved efficiency, higher quality of care, and better client outcomes. His story highlighted the importance of addressing nurse burnout as a systemic issue that requires holistic solutions and ongoing commitment.

Noah's impact started to spread across various levels of the healthcare system. His focus on enhancing nurses' working conditions ignited a broader discussion about the overall structure of healthcare workforces. He highlighted the significance of a harmonious team where the responsibilities and demands of healthcare are distributed more fairly among doctors, nurses, and other healthcare professionals. This approach aimed to foster a more inclusive and egalitarian framework, leading to enhanced collaboration and quality of care for clients.

Noah started to engage with the community alongside his work in the hospital system. He orchestrated community events and seminars to enlighten the public about nurses' vital role in healthcare and their challenges. These rallies generated widespread attention and community backing for the cause of nurse welfare.

Noah's initiatives also caught the attention of technology firms, leading to collaborations that explored technological solutions to reduce nurse workload. This involved the development of sophisticated client monitoring systems, administrative tools powered by artificial intelligence, and various other digital health technologies. These technologies aimed to streamline routine tasks, allowing nurses to prioritise client care over managerial duties.

Noah's successful lobbying efforts established a nationwide network of nurse advocates. This network offers a platform for nurses from different locations to exchange ideas, strategies, and achievements in enhancing workplace environments. It also served as a cohesive voice advocating national healthcare policy and reforms.

The story of Noah's endeavours to tackle nurse burnout at Mercy Mwongozo Hospital and other locations became a captivating illustration of successful lobbying and leadership. His journey showcased the power of concentrated efforts to bring about meaningful transformation and improve nurses' working conditions.

Noah's activities inspired and impacted others, serving as a worldwide role model for healthcare systems. His efforts demonstrated a commitment to cultivating a hospital environment that encourages and appreciates nurses. Noah's work highlighted nurses' important role in the healthcare system and emphasised the need for supportive environments that prioritise client well-being.

Noah advocated for a healthcare model recognising the interconnectedness of staff well-being and client care. His work highlighted the importance of addressing the challenges nurses face, not just for their gain but also for the betterment of the healthcare system. Noah's journey highlighted the significance of unwavering dedication and ingenuity in tackling the challenging problem of nurse burnout, guaranteeing that the healthcare staff receives the necessary support, maintains good health, and delivers optimal care.

Noah's activities have influenced policy formulation at various healthcare facilities. Hospitals and healthcare organisations started reconsidering their policies, prioritising efforts to reduce nurse burnout. All integral components were revamping nurse-to-client ratios, restructuring shift patterns to prioritise adequate rest, and implementing robust support systems for nurses navigating challenging and emotionally taxing situations.

In addition, Noah's campaign emphasised the importance of providing nurses with opportunities for career growth. He strongly supported programs that offered continuous learning, specialisation, and career advancement in nursing. These programs aimed to enhance the skills and engagement of nurses, ensuring their ongoing motivation and involvement in their work.

Noah understood the crucial significance of fostering a supportive community within the workplace to further his goal of assisting nurses. He actively encouraged the establishment of nurse-led committees focused on wellness and professional development. These committees offered a platform for nurses to voice their concerns, dialogue about their experiences, and contribute to the decision-making processes related to their work environment and professional growth.

Noah was crucial in fostering partnerships between healthcare institutions and academic scholars. These collaborations centred around researching nursing burnout, its underlying factors, and practical strategies for prevention. The research findings provided valuable insights that significantly impacted policies and practices aimed at reducing burnout and enhancing the work environment for nurses.

The story of Noah's tireless efforts to address nurse burnout resonated deeply within the healthcare industry, inspiring numerous other organisations to follow suit. His endeavours shed light on the crucial significance of prioritising the well-being of healthcare personnel and clients.

Noah's initiatives continued to inspire and impact people worldwide, serving as a model for healthcare organisations around the globe. He was committed to cultivating a healthcare culture that appreciates and uplifts nurses. Noah's efforts were a powerful reminder of the importance of acknowledging and tackling nurses' challenges.

Noah's book had a significant impact on enhancing working conditions for nurses and elevating the overall standard of healthcare. His journey underscored the importance of enduring, encouraging, and fostering work environments in healthcare settings. Noah's research highlighted the importance of a comprehensive approach to address nurse burnout. This involves implementing policy changes, establishing support networks, and fostering a culture that values and addresses the needs of nurses. His unwavering commitment to this cause led to positive advancements, guaranteeing that nurses received the necessary support and recognition.

CHAPTER 31

Sophia's Community Contribution

Sophia, a dedicated Mercy Mwongozo Hospital healthcare professional, has devoted her energy to enhancing healthcare in underserved areas. Her passion for community health arose from a deep belief in equal access to quality healthcare for all, regardless of their background or economic status. Sophia's community health programs have yielded significant outcomes, positively impacting the lives of numerous individuals.

She took a community-centred approach, strongly emphasising comprehending the residents' distinct needs and concerns. Sophia started by actively participating in extensive community outreach initiatives, reaching out to individuals, localities, and community groups to build trust and comprehensively understand the community's health requirements.

Sophia's main focus was setting up mobile health clinics in communities lacking sufficient healthcare access. These clinics provided essential medical services, including health screenings, vaccines, and health education. The healthcare professionals from Mercy Mwongozo Hospital operated the mobile clinics, providing medical care directly to needy individuals.

Sophia recognised the importance of education in improving community well-being. She organised health education workshops on nutrition, chronic illness management, and preventative healthcare. These workshops were tailored to meet the community's specific needs and played a crucial role in empowering locals with the necessary knowledge to manage their health effectively.

Sophia focused on addressing the factors influencing health outcomes and providing direct healthcare services. She collaborated with local organisations to initiate programs tackling food insecurity, housing instability, and unemployment, significantly impacting community health.

The fruits of Sophia's labour became evident in the improved health statistics of the individuals she dedicated herself to helping. There has been a noticeable decrease in common preventable diseases and a rise in people actively engaging in regular health check-ups and preventive measures.

Sophia's involvement in community health activities enhanced Mercy Mwongozo Hospital's connection with the surrounding communities. The hospital was now seen as more than just a healthcare provider but an active contributor to the community's overall welfare.

Her achievements were acknowledged beyond the local community as well. Sophia has been invited to speak at several healthcare conferences and forums, where she has shared her insights and success stories from her community health programs. Her methods started replicating in other towns, leading to significant advancements in community healthcare.

Sophia's community health work at Mercy Mwongozo Hospital unfolded as a tale of impact, empowerment, and profound transformation. Her journey showcased the significant impact healthcare professionals can have by extending their care beyond the confines of hospitals and into the fabric of communities.

Sophia's actions continued to inspire and guide, showcasing the importance of community health engagement. Her initiatives showcased a solid commitment to an inclusive healthcare system supporting and uplifting marginalised communities. Sophia's endeavours were a powerful reminder of the importance of tackling community healthcare concerns and guaranteeing everyone access to high-quality healthcare. Her journey exemplified the significance of unwavering commitment and forward-thinking in community health, ensuring that the most marginalised individuals receive essential care and support.

Sophia's impact on the community went beyond the immediate medical effects. She fostered connections with local schools, companies, and non-profit organisations to promote community health. These collaborations centred on developing long-term health promotion programs to improve well-being, including physical exercise, mental health, and nutrition.

Her approach also involved educating community members to become advocates for health. Sophia trained local volunteers in primary health education and preventive care, enabling them to become community health ambassadors. This peer-led methodology proved highly effective in promoting health awareness and fostering positive health behaviours.

Appreciating the significance of lasting influence, Sophia orchestrated community health forums where residents could discuss health matters, exchange personal stories, and offer input on the healthcare services they received regularly. These forums fostered a stronger sense of ownership among community members and ensured that healthcare efforts aligned with their needs.

Sophia was also dedicated to integrating technological solutions to enhance community health outreach. She implemented telehealth services to facilitate remote consultations, catering to individuals facing mobility constraints or residing in remote areas. This technological application has played a crucial role in addressing disparities in healthcare access and ensuring more effective management of chronic illnesses.

Sophia's community health efforts significantly impacted her, decreasing emergency room visits and hospitalisations in the communities she served. This outcome enhanced the community's overall well-being and lessened the strain on hospital resources, demonstrating the effectiveness of proactive community health interventions.

Sophia's endeavours also influenced public policy. Her diligent work impacted local health policies, leading to more significant funding for community health programs and infrastructure. She advanced in local health committees, using her knowledge to develop policies that promote equitable healthcare access.

Sophia's narrative about her involvement in community health work at Mercy Mwongozo Hospital and beyond offered a captivating portrayal of how healthcare professionals can bring about significant transformations beyond the confines of conventional hospital environments. Her journey showcased the power of involving the community, promoting education, and fostering innovation to address public health challenges.

Sophia's actions were a model for effective community health engagement, inspiring and influencing others. Her endeavours showcased a commitment to a healthcare system that embraces inclusivity, takes proactive measures, and is attentive to the community's needs. Sophia's work demonstrated a strong belief in the power of healthcare practitioners to positively impact marginalised communities, contributing to the development of healthier and more resilient societies. Her unwavering commitment to community health highlighted the importance of holistic, community-focused strategies to address the complex healthcare needs of diverse populations.

Sophia's actions started to shape a sustainable community health paradigm that could be replicated in other regions. She meticulously crafted a comprehensive guide that delves into the intricate concepts and methodology behind her highly effective programs. This manual is valuable for healthcare professionals and organisations implementing community health programs. It provides a comprehensive guide and serves as a blueprint for success.

Her focus on proactive healthcare led to the implementation of health screenings for the entire community. These screenings helped identify common health issues like diabetes, hypertension, and heart disease, which are prevalent in underprivileged communities. Recognising symptoms early led to prompt treatment, significantly improving overall health.

Sophia implemented mental health awareness programs as part of her comprehensive approach to addressing all facets of health. She facilitated workshops and support groups to reduce the stigma surrounding mental health and improve the accessibility of mental health services. These programs proved to be highly impactful as they addressed the often-overlooked issue of mental health in these communities, which was hindered by social stigma and limited resources.

Sophia deeply understood the importance of cultural sensitivity in healthcare delivery. She ensured that her programs were culturally relevant and respectful of the diverse backgrounds within the community. This approach fostered trust and enhanced the probability of healthcare advice being embraced and incorporated into everyday routines.

In addition, Sophia's work in community health started to generate scholarly interest. Universities and research institutions investigated the impact of her programs, generating crucial data that further validated her techniques. The research findings contributed to the improvement of her programs and provided academic evidence of the effectiveness of community-focused healthcare initiatives.

The success of Sophia's community health programs led to increased investment from both the public and commercial sectors. This funding allowed her to broaden her reach and offer a broader range of services, expanding her impact and reaching more people. Furthermore, it enabled the integration of cutting-edge healthcare technologies and resources.

Sophia's approach to community health involved implementing measures to improve environmental well-being. She understood the significance of creating a conducive environment for health and well-being. Consequently, she collaborated with environmental experts to address concerns like pollution, access to clean water, and safe housing, all of which directly impacted the well-being of community members.

Sophia's story of her involvement in community health work at Mercy Mwongozo Hospital and beyond is a testament to the power of empowerment, innovation, and a holistic approach to health. Her experience highlighted the importance of considering the broader factors that influence health and engaging communities in their healthcare, which can lead to notable advancements in public health.

Sophia's endeavours served as a source of inspiration and guidance for others, exemplifying comprehensive and inclusive approaches to community health. Her initiatives showcased a commitment to a healthcare system that extends beyond the clinical setting and into the fabric of communities. Sophia's work highlighted the importance of considering all aspects of health, such as physical, mental, environmental, and social factors, to promote proper health equity and community well-being.

Her unwavering dedication to community health underscores the importance of being flexible, culturally aware, and innovative in meeting communities' diverse and evolving needs. Sophia's work highlighted the importance of understanding and appreciating the distinct characteristics of different communities to carry out successful community health initiatives. Additionally, she emphasised the significance of empowering community members to participate actively in their well-being. Her journey became a blueprint for effective, empathetic, and sustainable community health initiatives, leading to a future where everyone can enjoy better health and fairness.

Sophia aims to create a more vibrant community that involves working closely with nearby educational institutions. She developed programs where healthcare personnel from Mercy Mwongozo Hospital, including herself, would go to schools to educate children and teenagers about health and wellness. The training programs covered many themes, including basic hygiene and nutrition, mental health awareness, and disease prevention. Sophia was determined to instil healthy habits in the younger generation from an early age, leading to positive long-term effects on community health.

Her commitment to community health also led to developing specialised programs for different population segments. She diligently arranged frequent health fairs for older people, providing screenings and health education tailored to their needs. She conducted workshops for parents and young families, offering valuable insights on pediatric health, nutrition, and developmental milestones.

Sophia understood the importance of addressing chronic diseases, which were widespread among the population, in her quest to offer comprehensive treatment. She established support groups and disease management programs for individuals with diabetes and heart disease. These programs incorporated knowledge of disease management, lifestyle enhancements, and medication adherence, significantly enhancing the client's quality of life.

Sophia also tried to integrate behavioural health into her community health programs. She understood the strong connection between physical and mental health. She enhanced the availability of counselling services and developed support systems focused on promoting mental well-being, managing stress, and developing coping strategies.

Sophia incorporated digital health technologies into her community programs, acknowledging the significant impact of technology on improving healthcare. These options encompass utilising health applications to monitor fitness and nutrition, telehealth services for consultations from a distance, and online health education platforms. These technological advancements expanded healthcare accessibility and facilitated continuous communication with community members.

Sophia's endeavours had a profound influence. The communities she served experienced significant improvements in their overall health indicators. There was a significant decrease in emergency room visits and a notable decline in rates of preventable diseases. The Mwongozo health awareness and habits of the community showed marked improvement.

Sophia's actions further contributed to fostering a stronger sense of community. People started coming together more often, not just for health-related events but also for activities that fostered a sense of community. The sense of community was crucial in sustaining health improvements and supporting each other on their health journeys.

Sophia's narrative about her involvement in community health work at Mercy Mwongozo Hospital is a testament to the impact of committed, empathetic, and forward-thinking healthcare endeavours. Her journey showcased the potential of proactive, community-centred healthcare to bring about significant and lasting improvements in public health.

Sophia's efforts continued to motivate and provide guidance, establishing the foundation for effective community health involvement. Her endeavours showcased a solid commitment to a healthcare system that is deeply integrated within the communities it serves. Sophia's efforts served as a powerful reminder of the crucial role that healthcare practitioners can play in treating illness, promoting health, preventing disease, and inspiring communities to take an active role in their health and well-being. Her unwavering dedication to community health was a guiding light, shedding light on the path toward a more enlightened and cohesive society.

Sophia's influence on community health started to extend beyond the local level, inspiring other healthcare practitioners and organisations to do the same. Her approach to community engagement and comprehensive treatment became a benchmark for exceptional community health programs. Healthcare professionals from all corners of the country flocked to her programs, filled with enthusiasm to acquire and implement her techniques in their respective fields.

Sophia has been honoured with numerous awards and accolades from esteemed health organisations and community groups, acknowledging her exceptional contributions. These accolades fueled her drive to expand her sphere of influence and make a meaningful difference. She actively engaged in discussions surrounding policy, advocating for more significant financial support for community health initiatives, with a particular focus on underserved regions.

Sophia played a crucial role in establishing a network of community health professionals. These individuals, who often resided in the communities they served, were trained to deliver essential healthcare services and act as intermediaries between the community and healthcare professionals. This network significantly broadened the reach of healthcare services, ensuring that individuals in even the most remote or isolated areas could access essential care.

Sophia's projects have also started to incorporate concerns about environmental health. She collaborated with local governments and environmental organisations to tackle pressing concerns such as clean water access, pollution, and safe housing, recognising the profound impact these issues had on the health and well-being of community members.

Sophia pioneered utilising community health data to inform and enhance her programs. Through careful analysis of health trends and outcomes, she made informed decisions and adapted her programs to serve the community's evolving needs better. This approach ensured that her programs stayed up-to-date, impactful, and streamlined.

The success of her efforts led to increased funding and support from healthcare institutions, local companies, and philanthropic organisations. This support allowed Sophia to broaden her endeavours, providing supplementary programs and reaching a more significant population segment.

Sophia's work in community health at Mercy Mwongozo Hospital and beyond is a remarkable tale of dedication, creativity, and community empowerment. Her experience highlighted the critical role that healthcare professionals could have in positively impacting the community.

Sophia's endeavours have consistently inspired and provided guidance, serving as a model for engaging with global community health. Her endeavours showcased a commitment to a healthcare system that proactively engages with and uplifts its members. Sophia's endeavours were a powerful testament to the importance of comprehensive, community-focused approaches in addressing public health issues and enhancing community members' overall health and welfare. Her unwavering dedication to community health exemplified the profound influence that healthcare professionals can have on public health and the overall well-being of communities.

CHAPTER 32

Integrating Technology and Empathy

Emma, a forward-thinking healthcare expert at Mercy Mwongozo Hospital, embarked on an innovative mission to integrate technology with compassionate care. She proposed utilising artificial intelligence (AI) to enhance client care while preserving the crucial human element in healthcare. Her innovative idea revolutionised how Mercy Mwongozo cared for clients by integrating artificial intelligence with compassion.

The project's focal point revolved around developing an AI-driven system to assist healthcare professionals in client management. This system utilised sophisticated algorithms to analyse client data, aiding in the timely identification of potential health risks and providing guidance for treatment choices. Emma was focused on ensuring that this technology worked alongside, rather than substituting, the human aspects of care.

Emma taught the hospital personnel the AI system through workshops and training sessions. These workshops aim to acquaint personnel with the technology and address any concerns regarding its implementation. Emma emphasised the importance of the AI system as a complement to their skills rather than a substitute for their expertise or compassion.

Emma's project also focused on utilising artificial intelligence to tailor client care, which proved crucial. The system has the potential to acquire knowledge from each client's distinct health histories and preferences, enabling healthcare providers to offer more personalised treatment and care plans. This customisation led to greater satisfaction and engagement among clients in their healthcare.

Emma was also focused on ensuring that the AI system was easy to use and accessible to all. She worked closely with the technology team to develop a user-friendly interface for healthcare professionals and clients. The focus on usability facilitated the seamless integration of this technology into everyday healthcare procedures.

Emma devised a client feedback method to find a harmonious blend of technology and empathy. Clients were encouraged to provide feedback on their interactions with the AI system, ensuring their perspectives were considered in the technology's ongoing development.

Emma's project had a significant impact. The AI system enhanced healthcare delivery efficiency by reducing administrative burdens on healthcare personnel, allowing them to allocate more time to delivering direct client care. It also improved precision and efficiency in diagnosis, resulting in better client outcomes.

Emma's innovative approach to combining technology and empathy in healthcare gained recognition beyond Mercy Mwongozo Hospital. She has been invited to speak at healthcare technology conferences and forums, where she has shared her insights on how technology can enhance, rather than diminish, the human aspects of healthcare.

Emma's work at Mercy Mwongozo Hospital exemplified a remarkable blend of technology and compassionate care, resulting in a story of healthcare innovation, balance, and foresight. Her narrative underscored the potential benefits of incorporating intelligent technology into healthcare, enhancing both the quality and efficiency of care, all while preserving the essential elements of empathy and human connection.

Emma's endeavours remained a source of inspiration and exerted a significant impact, laying the foundation for the seamless integration of healthcare technology in the years to come. Her work showcased a solid commitment to leveraging technological advancements in healthcare to enhance client care, all while maintaining a deep sense of compassion and empathy. Emma's dedication highlighted the profound impact of technology on healthcare, emphasising its role in enhancing and augmenting human interaction rather than supplanting it. Her steadfast commitment to achieving this equilibrium paved the path for a new era in healthcare, where technology and compassion harmoniously work together to provide optimal client care.

Emma's idea started to come together as she incorporated input from healthcare professionals and individuals receiving care. She understood the importance of continuously enhancing the AI system to meet the evolving demands of healthcare delivery. She collaborated with technology experts to develop advanced features, including natural language processing capabilities. These enhancements enabled the system to respond to client requests in a more human-like manner.

To achieve a harmonious blend of technology and compassion, Emma integrated virtual reality (VR) simulations into the training of healthcare professionals. These simulations offered a captivating experience that helped staff grasp the effective utilisation of AI tools while maintaining a compassionate approach to client care.

The AI system also included a component that monitored the clients' psychological state. The technology could use sentiment analysis to provide healthcare providers with insights into individuals who may be experiencing heightened stress or anxiety. This would enable timely interventions with a personalised approach.

Emma also explored the use of AI to enhance client education and engagement. Clients were provided tailored instructional content to meet their diagnoses and treatment plans. This empowered individuals to understand their health better and take a more proactive role in their healthcare, leading to enhanced health outcomes and increased client independence.

The medical community acknowledged and endorsed Emma's efforts as the project gained momentum. The fusion of artificial intelligence and compassionate care was noteworthy in client-centered healthcare. Emma's idea started to shape the perspectives of other hospitals and healthcare institutions regarding technology in healthcare.

Emma's narrative of integrating technology with compassionate care has continued to be a symbol of innovation and empathy in the healthcare field. Her story showcased the immense power of technology to transform healthcare when used with wisdom and in conjunction with the human elements of care.

Emma's drive and ingenuity inspired and shaped a new standard for incorporating technology in healthcare. Her work showcased a deep commitment to a healthcare system that embraces technological advancements while upholding principles of empathy and compassion. Emma's research showcased the remarkable potential of combining technology and human care, illustrating a future where healthcare quality is enhanced by technology while still preserving the personal touch. Her steadfast dedication to this vision paved the path for a healthcare system that is more streamlined, impactful, and empathetic, where technology and compassion work together to enhance client care and results.

Emma's project began to shape people's views on technology in healthcare. The remarkable achievement of integrating AI with compassionate care at Mercy Mwongozo Hospital demonstrates technology's immense potential in enhancing the human elements of healthcare. The AI solution improved clinical decision-making, streamlined administrative processes, and allowed healthcare personnel to dedicate more time to client engagement and care.

Emma collaborated with cybersecurity experts to ensure the AI system met the necessary security standards and complied with healthcare regulations, demonstrating a solid commitment to safeguarding client privacy and protecting data. She recognised the significance of client trust and ensured all technical implementations upheld and defended client privacy.

Emma delved into the role of AI in chronic disease management as the research advanced. The system was enhanced to constantly monitor clients with chronic diseases, offering healthcare providers up-to-date data that could be utilised to modify treatment programs proactively. This approach not only improved client outcomes but also empowered individuals to actively engage in managing their health.

Emma also recognised the potential of AI to improve healthcare accessibility for marginalised communities. She utilised the AI system and initiated a pilot program to deliver healthcare services to underserved and distant regions. This program employed telehealth and remote monitoring technology to provide medical consultations and ongoing care, thus eliminating geographical barriers to healthcare access.

The project profoundly influenced the education of upcoming healthcare professionals. Emma collaborated with medical and nursing schools to integrate AI and technology training into healthcare. This training ensured that new healthcare professionals were well-prepared to work efficiently with emerging technologies, arming them for a modern era of healthcare delivery.

Emma's narrative of integrating technology and compassionate care has consistently motivated and transformed the healthcare industry. Her journey showcased the power of compassion and deep insight into client needs, resulting in groundbreaking healthcare advancements.

Emma's project has significantly influenced and set a standard for incorporating technology in healthcare. Her work showcased a commitment to a healthcare system that effectively utilises technology to enhance client care, all while upholding a strong focus on empathy and compassion. Emma's effort showcased the seamless synergy that can be achieved in healthcare when technology and human compassion come together. Her unwavering dedication to achieving this equilibrium opened the way for a more refined comprehension of how technology can treat and nurture clients. Emma's journey highlighted the importance of ongoing innovation; design focused on clients, and empathetic implementation in incorporating technology into healthcare. Her work has inspired the future of healthcare, where technology and compassion come together to create a more impactful, streamlined, and compassionate healthcare journey.

Emma's dedication started to have a profound impact on the delivery of healthcare and the public perception of it. The fusion of AI and compassionate care has begun to alleviate numerous clients' concerns regarding advancements in healthcare technology. They started to view technology as a tool that, when utilised with empathy, could significantly enhance their care experience rather than an impersonal entity.

Emma utilised advanced machine learning techniques to continuously enhance the AI system, enabling it to acquire knowledge and adjust based on every client interaction. Their adaptability makes AI recommendations increasingly personalised and precise, improving treatment plans and client outcomes.

Emma also understood the importance of continuous feedback from healthcare professionals and clients in improving the AI system. She established regular review sessions to analyse feedback and make adjustments. This collaborative approach ensured the system aligned with its users' authentic needs and expectations.

The success of Emma's project started to attract global recognition. Healthcare organisations from all over the globe have shown keen interest in her work and are eager to gain insights into implementing similar systems in their respective settings. Emma's project had a significant global impact, leading to advancements in healthcare technology and improving client care globally.

Emma also started exploring the potential of AI in personalised medicine. She envisioned a future where AI could play a pivotal role in developing customised treatment strategies tailored to an individual's genetic profile, lifestyle choices, and medical background. This approach could revolutionise therapy's effectiveness and enhance client care quality.

Emma's story of combining technology and compassionate care has consistently stood out as an innovative example in healthcare. Her journey uncovered the immense potential of utilising technology to enhance the efficiency of healthcare delivery and foster stronger connections between clients and carers.

Emma's efforts have consistently motivated and directed, leading to a fresh era of healthcare technology. Her work showcased a commitment to a healthcare system that prioritises compassion and puts clients at the centre while embracing technological advancements. Emma's project showcased the remarkable progress that can be achieved in healthcare through empathy and deep comprehension of client requirements. Her steadfast dedication to this vision ushered in a new era in healthcare, where technology serves as a conduit, fortifying the connection between clients and healthcare professionals and enhancing health outcomes and experiences. Emma's experience was a guiding light, shedding light on a more empathetic, efficient, and technologically advanced healthcare future.

CHAPTER 33

A World Without Borders

David, an experienced healthcare professional at Mercy Mwongozo Hospital, acknowledged the global nature of contemporary health concerns. His commitment to a healthier planet inspired him to participate in the pandemic prevention program. His research aimed to decrease the chances of future pandemics through global cooperation, vigilance, and creativity.

The program was created with the understanding that a health issue in one place can have far-reaching consequences in our interconnected world. David started by establishing partnerships with healthcare organisations, governments, and scholars from around the globe. These collaborations focused on sharing knowledge, resources, and techniques for identifying, averting, and addressing potential pandemic threats.

David had a wide-ranging role in the program. He supervised efforts to develop extensive surveillance systems to identify early signs of outbreaks. This involved merging data from various sources, such as healthcare institutions, laboratories, and social media, to track and analyse disease patterns.

David focused on developing worldwide response capabilities alongside surveillance. During health emergencies, he concentrated on enhancing international communication and fostering cooperation. Developing protocols for efficient information exchange, mobilising resources, and coordinating intervention plans were all integral to this endeavour.

David advocated for increased research into the development of infectious diseases, highlighting the importance of prevention. He supported efforts to gain a deeper understanding of the origins of illnesses, how they spread, and effective methods to control and prevent them. This research was crucial in developing vaccinations, therapies, and preventive measures.

David also acknowledged the significance of involving the community in pandemic preparedness. He initiated public awareness campaigns to educate individuals about the importance of hygiene, vaccination, and promptly reporting early symptoms. These programs were designed to inspire individuals to actively participate in mitigating the spread of diseases.

As the program gained momentum, David's hard work started to pay off. Surveillance systems have advanced in both sophistication and effectiveness in detecting potential threats. Global partnerships led to faster and more synchronised reactions to health crises. In addition, the research activities resulted in valuable insights that contributed to the development of novel prevention and treatment strategies.

The narrative surrounding David's involvement in the program became one of forward-thinking, collaboration, and a sense of global accountability. His tour highlighted the importance of international cooperation in combating pandemics and the interconnectedness of health worldwide.

David's actions continued to inspire and influence, serving as a model for active engagement in global health. His work exemplified a commitment to a society where borders do not determine health and safety boundaries. David's actions highlighted the importance of worldwide collaboration and awareness in preventing future pandemics. His steadfast dedication to this cause propelled advancements toward a brighter, more prosperous future for everyone.

David's involvement began to spur significant progress in global health security. His advocacy for a collaborative approach led to establishing more robust networks between nations, enhancing the ability to address health challenges together. These networks facilitated the exchange of information and the sharing of resources and knowledge, which is crucial in rapidly containing outbreaks.

David prioritised enhancing the capabilities in susceptible areas as a testament to his dedication to fostering a robust worldwide health framework. He understood that the strength of the global health system relied on its most vulnerable components. In pursuit of this goal, he passionately advocated for initiatives that enhanced healthcare systems in disadvantaged areas by providing training, equipment, and assistance to local healthcare professionals. This work equipped these regions to handle local outbreaks more efficiently and reduced the chances of regional crises escalating into global concerns.

David played a crucial role in shaping ethical principles for international health responses. During times of crisis, he advocated for policies that promoted fair and equal access to healthcare resources, medicines, and vaccines. His work highlighted the belief that every person deserves access to proper healthcare and safety, regardless of geographical location.

David also acknowledged the potential of advancing technologies to enhance pandemic preparedness. He collaborated with technology businesses and entrepreneurs to develop innovative solutions such as AI-driven outbreak prediction models, mobile health apps for real-time illness monitoring, and virtual healthcare worker training platforms. These technological advancements have contributed significantly to the early detection and effective management of health issues.

As its popularity increased, so did its influence. The program was instrumental in preventing local outbreaks from turning into global catastrophes. These achievements showcased the program's effectiveness and emphasised the significance of proactive and collaborative international health policies. David's efforts in preventing the pandemic showcased the power of working together to address global health issues. His experience highlighted the critical significance of forward-thinking, teamwork, and creativity in building a world that can withstand health risks.

David's endeavours sparked and directed, ushering in a new era of worldwide engagement in health. His work exemplified a commitment to a future where the collective responsibility for health is prioritised, leaving no one susceptible to the devastating impacts of pandemics. David's endeavours were a powerful testament to the potential of cooperation and ingenuity in shaping a more secure and prosperous future for all. His steadfast dedication to this objective has paved the way for ongoing advancements in global health security, inspiring others to join the mission of creating a world without boundaries.

David's strong belief in global unity against health dangers led him to passionately advocate for more comprehensive measures that surpassed national policy and individual initiatives. He championed a global health framework that integrated economic, social, and environmental issues, acknowledging the interconnectedness of health determinants and the need for a comprehensive approach. He started collaborating with leaders from various sectors, such as agriculture, education, and trade, to tackle the underlying factors that impacted health. These alliances aimed to address health hazards at their source, promoting sustainable farming techniques to prevent foodborne infections and advocating for higher air quality standards to reduce respiratory disorders.

David emphasised the importance of cultural knowledge in global health initiatives. He understood the significance of acknowledging and comprehending cultural differences in effectively communicating and implementing health policies among diverse groups. He strongly supported integrating cultural studies into healthcare professional training, recognising its potential to enhance its effectiveness in international contexts. In addition, David's research shifted its focus toward the psychological aspects of global health concerns. He advocated for mental health treatment not only for affected individuals but also for healthcare staff who experienced significant stress and trauma while handling outbreaks. He strongly emphasised the importance of incorporating mental health into the global response to health crises.

David understood the importance of fostering innovation in healthcare delivery as he worked towards building a robust global health system. He strongly supported the establishment of mobile health clinics, telemedicine, and other methods of remote healthcare that could provide services in distant areas. These advancements played a crucial role in regions with inadequate healthcare systems or during times of restricted movements, such as during disease outbreaks.

David has also dedicated his efforts to enhancing global health education. He created exchange programs for healthcare professionals and students to gain practical experience in different healthcare environments across the globe. These programs encouraged a heightened understanding of global health challenges and the open sharing of ideas and proven methods. As it gained popularity, it became a model for international health cooperation. The program's effectiveness was highlighted in global forums, and other governments and organisations replicated its methods. David's commitment to fostering a collaborative approach to health security ignited a global movement towards greater unity and effectiveness in health measures.

David's narrative of global health security transformed into a captivating account of foresight, cooperation, and resilience. His experience showcased the immense impact of working together to create a more sustainable and thriving planet. It highlighted the difficulties and intricacies of global health and the significance of continuous commitment, creativity, and unity.

David's endeavours profoundly influenced and served as a source of inspiration for others, playing a pivotal role in shaping the future of global health engagement. His endeavours showcased a commitment to a global vision where the importance of health security is universally recognised, and proactive measures are taken to safeguard the welfare of individuals, irrespective of their location or situation. David's endeavours were a remarkable testament to the belief that, as a society, we can overcome health obstacles by coming together, being proactive, and showing compassion. His steadfast dedication to this cause has propelled advancements in global health security, motivating others to unite in guaranteeing health for everyone, both presently and in the years to come.

David's influence in shaping global health policy became more significant as his involvement with "A World Without Borders" expanded. He established himself as a respected advisor to international health organisations, guiding global health preparedness and response. His contributions helped advance the development of tactics that were effective, fair, and considerate of the needs of diverse individuals. He also began contemplating the impact of technology on enhancing global health surveillance and response. David passionately advocated for the establishment of a worldwide health information network. This platform would enable governments and organisations to exchange health data, research findings, and resources securely and efficiently. This network strives to enhance real-time communication and collaboration, allowing the global health community to be more agile and ready to respond to catastrophes.

David understood the crucial role of solid communities in preventing pandemics. Alongside his policy and technology efforts, he dedicated his efforts to community-based programs that enhance local capabilities in identifying and addressing health issues. These programs empowered communities to actively participate in safeguarding their well-being through initiatives focused on preventing illnesses and promoting good health.

David's study highlighted the significance of establishing sustainable funding systems for global health projects. He collaborated with financial institutions, governments, and philanthropic organisations to develop funding mechanisms to ensure continuous and sufficient investment in global health security. This support was crucial in maintaining and enhancing the infrastructure, resources, and programs necessary to prevent and address health hazards.

David's efforts have a global influence, reaching people from all walks of life. Nations that adopted the strategies and advancements outlined in "A World Without Borders" experienced enhanced preparedness and expedited, better-coordinated reactions to health crises. These triumphs reinforced David's belief in the importance of a unified global effort to combat pandemics. As David gained traction, he continued to advocate for a worldwide health ethic of continuous learning and improvement. He emphasised the importance of studying and analysing every health crisis to improve future reactions. This involved conducting evaluations after crises, sharing insights acquired, and adjusting strategies and policies as necessary.

David's narrative on pandemic prevention and global health security is a powerful testament to the immense potential of working together, staying well-informed, and taking proactive measures to address health issues. His journey demonstrated the power of dedication, creativity, and international collaboration in creating a safer and healthier world.

David's endeavours continued to serve as a source of inspiration and guidance, establishing the foundation for forthcoming global health endeavours. His work exemplified a commitment to creating a global society where everyone has equal access to necessary healthcare and treatment regardless of location. David's endeavours were a powerful reminder of the intricate relationship between health and the collective duty to protect it. His unwavering dedication to this objective drove advancements in global health by inspiring collaborative effort and fostering a spirit of unity and readiness in the face of health threats.

CHAPTER 34

Lina's Legacy

Lina, a respected educator and innovator at Mercy Mwongozo Hospital, has been leading the way in enhancing nursing education for a significant period. Her dedication and innovative approaches have improved nursing education and practice. "Lina's Legacy" gained a reputation for excellence and innovation in nursing education as her unique methods garnered increased recognition.

Her journey started with a clear and powerful vision: establishing an educational setting where nurses were proficient professionals, empathetic carers, and analytical problem solvers. Lina developed a program highlighting the importance of empathy, ethics, and communication in addition to rigorous scientific training. This approach ensured that graduates were well-equipped to tackle the intricate demands of contemporary healthcare.

Lina was a strong proponent of simulation-based learning. She developed state-of-the-art simulation labs where students can practice clinical skills in a secure and supervised environment. These simulations were designed to replicate real-life situations, helping students refine their decision-making and problem-solving skills. This practical, immersive learning experience has a profound effect, leading to nursing graduates who are more self-assured and skilled.

Given the rapid advancements in healthcare, Lina highlighted the importance of continuous learning. She developed continuing education programs to ensure nurses stay informed about the latest advancements in healthcare innovation and client care methods. The focus on ongoing professional development has significantly elevated the standard of nursing practice at Mercy Mwongozo and other institutions.

Lina's dedication to integrating interdisciplinary learning into the nursing curriculum was groundbreaking. She facilitated collaborative training sessions with students from medical, pharmacy, and social work backgrounds, fostering a team-oriented approach to client care. Nursing students received comprehensive training that prepared them to excel in the ever-evolving healthcare field, where collaboration is critical.

Other institutions started paying attention as news of Lina's innovative strategies spread. She was invited to share her insights and expertise at prestigious nursing conferences nationally and internationally. Her work significantly impacted nursing education as more institutions embraced her ideas and methodology.

Lina's exceptional achievements were acknowledged with numerous prestigious accolades and awards from prominent healthcare and educational institutions. These awards recognised her significant contributions to nursing education and her efforts to enhance healthcare through improved nurse training and preparedness.

Lina's story of transforming nursing education at Mercy Mwongozo Hospital is a testament to her vision, unwavering commitment, and lasting impact. Her experience highlighted the profound impact of innovative educational methods and underscored the vital contribution of nurses in the healthcare system.

Lina's initiatives continued to inspire and guide, setting a forward-thinking and client-focused standard for nursing education. Her work showcased a solid commitment to educating nurses with clinical expertise, compassion, and readiness to navigate the ever-evolving healthcare industry. Lina's legacy was a powerful testament to the importance of pushing the boundaries of nursing education, continuously expanding knowledge, and fostering collaboration across disciplines. Her profound influence had a lasting effect on the nursing field, guaranteeing that the care provided by nurses was of exceptional calibre, characterised by empathy and comprehension.

Lina's impact expanded as her groundbreaking educational methods were embraced by nursing programs worldwide. Her unique approach established a standard by which modern nursing education was measured. Lina's teaching methods were highly regarded by institutions seeking to enhance their nursing programs, as they were thorough and focused on the needs of the students.

Lina's influence extended beyond the confines of the classroom, as evidenced by the positive healthcare outcomes achieved by her students in the communities they served. Graduates of her program received high accolades for their exceptional client care, sharp analytical skills, and seamless collaboration within diverse teams. Their expertise and empathy significantly impacted client satisfaction and the overall quality of healthcare.

Lina's guidance and example inspired aspiring nurse educators. She cultivated a community of educators who shared her passion for enhancing the quality and creativity of nursing education. She fostered a culture of ongoing education and advancement among her colleagues, utilising workshops, mentorship programs, and collaborative initiatives.

She had a profound impact on the field of nursing education research. Lina collaborated with academic researchers to explore the outcomes of her teaching methods, offering substantial data that contributed to the improvement and validation of her approach.

The findings of this study contributed to the increasing body of evidence supporting the effectiveness of her innovative strategies.

Lina's methods gained widespread recognition, establishing her as a leading advocate for the nursing field. She leveraged her position to highlight nurses' crucial role in healthcare and champion more significant investment in nursing education and professional growth. Her activism brought awareness to the needs and issues of the nursing profession, influencing legislative and financial decisions.

Lina's work in nursing education at Mercy Mwongozo Hospital and elsewhere is a testament to the impact of dedicated and creative teaching. Her story has inspired countless educators and healthcare workers to pursue excellence, innovation, and empathy.

Lina's endeavours continued to have a profound impact, serving as a source of inspiration and setting a precedent for the future of nursing education. Her work showcased a commitment to a highly skilled, adaptable, and genuinely caring nursing profession. Lina's impact was profound, propelling nursing education to strive for more outstanding excellence. Her enduring impact ensured that future nurses would possess the necessary knowledge, skills, and compassion to provide optimal client care in a constantly evolving healthcare landscape.

Lina's influence on nursing education brought about a significant transformation across healthcare facilities. The significance of highly skilled and empathetic nursing staff in client care and health outcomes has increased. Hospitals and healthcare facilities started investing more in their nursing staff, acknowledging nurses' crucial role in client care and providing avenues for professional development.

This cultural shift also influenced the way clients viewed their care. As nurses took on a more significant role in healthcare delivery, clients started to see them not only as carers but as essential contributors to their health journey. Lina's focus on effective communication and compassionate care in nursing fostered deeper connections between clients and their healthcare providers, resulting in a greater emphasis on personalised client care.

Lina embarked on a thorough exploration of the possibilities offered by cutting-edge technology in nursing education, driven by her unwavering commitment to achieving the highest standards. She acknowledged the potential of digital technologies, simulation, and virtual reality to enhance the learning experience by creating a more immersive and participatory environment for students. These technological advancements have facilitated more realistic and diverse teaching experiences, better-equipping students with the complexities of modern healthcare.

Lina's unwavering commitment to advancing nursing education has driven her to focus on addressing pressing global health issues. She incorporated international health concepts into her curriculum to ensure her students understood the broader health and healthcare delivery perspective. Her graduates were well-prepared to navigate diverse environments and make meaningful contributions to enhancing global health rather than solely focusing on local efforts.

Her work challenged the conventional boundaries that separated different healthcare disciplines. Lina advocated for a holistic approach to healthcare education, encouraging collaboration and knowledge-sharing among students from various health professions. This interprofessional education fostered a collaborative atmosphere in clinical practice, leading to enhanced client care that is comprehensive and well-coordinated.

Lina's expertise gained widespread recognition, leading to numerous invitations to guide nursing education programs across the globe. Her guidance was sought by institutions looking to modernise their curriculum and approach. Lina's influence extended beyond her institution, significantly impacting nursing education worldwide.

Lina's work in nursing education is a captivating narrative of impact, enthusiasm, and forward-thinking guidance. Her story showcased the remarkable influence that one individual can wield over an entire field and, in fact, the standard of healthcare worldwide.

Lina's activities inspired and guided others, setting a solid example for nursing education and professional growth. Her work showcased a strong commitment to educating nurses with expertise, proficiency, compassion, flexibility, and readiness to address the evolving challenges of healthcare. Lina's legacy highlighted the importance of continuous learning, innovation, and empathy in nursing education. Her lasting influence ensured that future nurses would be highly prepared to provide clients with global, empathetic, skilled, and meticulous care. Her forward-thinking mindset and unwavering dedication laid the foundation for a future where nursing education and practice thrive through ongoing growth, teamwork, and a relentless focus on client welfare.

Lina's influence started to make waves in the regulatory aspects of nursing education. She was accrediting theories, and professional nursing organisations recognised and embraced her innovative and holistic approaches in their standards and recommendations. As a result, her techniques gained wider acceptance, guaranteeing that future nurses would be trained in programs emphasising technical skills, empathy, critical thinking, and interprofessional teamwork.

Lina's profile skyrocketed, and she became a highly sought-after speaker and respected figure in the healthcare industry. She used this platform to passionately advocate for causes that deeply resonated with her, including the significance of mental health for healthcare professionals, the imperative of equitable healthcare access, and the pivotal role of nurses in shaping the future of healthcare. Her voice influenced public opinion and policy on these critical subjects.

Lina redirected her focus towards the mentorship of nurse educators as a testament to her unwavering dedication to enhancing nursing education. She established a mentorship program that connected seasoned educators with those starting in the field. This program helped spread her teaching methods and ensured that the core values of empathy, client-centred care, and lifelong learning were imparted to future educators and, through them, to countless nursing students.

Lina's work made a significant impression on the research community as well. Researchers were intrigued by her innovative techniques and impressive results, prompting them to conduct studies on the outcomes of her comprehensive approach to nursing education. The results showcased enduring improvements in client care, nurse contentment, and overall healthcare excellence, offering concrete proof to support Lina's approaches and principles.

In addition, Lina's work started to impact healthcare policy. Policymakers began to appreciate her support for nursing and innovative teaching techniques as essential elements of a robust healthcare system. This recognition led to additional funding for nursing education, enhanced support for nursing students, and more significant investment in the necessary tools and technology for effective nursing instruction.

Lina's story continued to evolve, showcasing the immense impact of visionary leadership in nursing education. Her journey showcased the profound influence that an individual's commitment and creativity can have on an entire field and the welfare and prosperity of global communities.

Lina's ideas sparked inspiration and profoundly impacted others, setting a high bar for excellence and innovation in nursing education. Her work exemplified a commitment to a future where nurses play a vital role in healthcare, not only as the foundation but also as the essence of it. Lina's impact on nursing education has been profound, inspiring a constant pursuit of greater empathy, excellence, and creativity. Her lasting influence ensured that future nurses would be equipped to handle the challenges of a constantly evolving healthcare environment with knowledge, empathy, and an unwavering commitment to client well-being.

CHAPTER 35

Aisha's Achievements

Aisha, a passionate healthcare professional at Mercy Mwongozo Hospital, has always strongly advocated for promoting diversity and inclusion in the healthcare field. Her innovative diversity program was designed to tackle the disparities and challenges marginalised groups face in the healthcare system. As her program yielded tangible results, it became strongly associated with advancements in healthcare and fostering inclusiveness.

Her program started by providing comprehensive training for healthcare personnel on cultural competency, sensitivity, and the importance of diversity in healthcare. This program sought to foster understanding and appreciation for clients' diverse backgrounds and unique needs, ensuring that every client received culturally sensitive care tailored to their circumstances.

Aisha also focused on recruiting and retention strategies to foster a more diverse healthcare workforce. She worked closely with human resources to establish policies that promoted recruiting individuals from various cultural, ethnic, and socioeconomic backgrounds. The diverse workforce at Mercy Mwongozo brought a wide range of perspectives and backgrounds, enhancing the quality of service.

Aisha's diversity program encompassed a range of initiatives, including community outreach programs and comprehensive staff training and recruitment efforts. She worked closely with community leaders and organisations to gain a deeper understanding of the distinct health needs of different groups. These collaborations helped customise healthcare services to meet the needs of each community better, resulting in improved responsiveness and success.

Aisha's program had a profound effect. Client satisfaction levels among underrepresented groups significantly increased, indicating that clients felt greater understanding, respect, and quality care. Healthcare workers also noted a heightened knowledge and proficiency in addressing cultural and individual differences, leading to a more personalised and compassionate approach to client care.

In addition, Aisha's endeavours led to increased fairness in healthcare. Her program tackled the systemic barriers that hindered healthcare access and quality for marginalised communities. Aisha's program addressed obstacles to improving health outcomes, ensuring equal opportunities for all clients to achieve optimal health.

Aisha's accomplishments in her diversity program were acknowledged beyond Mercy Mwongozo Hospital. Other organisations started seeking guidance from her program on fostering diversity and inclusivity in healthcare. Aisha has been invited to speak at conferences and seminars, where she has shared her insights and strategies for promoting a more inclusive healthcare environment.

Aisha's journey in her diversity program at Mercy Mwongozo Hospital unfolded as a story of growth, empathy, and appreciation. Her experience highlighted the significant impact a commitment to diversity and inclusion can have on the quality of care and the well-being of clients and healthcare providers.

Aisha's initiatives have consistently served as a source of inspiration and influence, demonstrating a blueprint for healthcare institutions to embrace and celebrate diversity. Her endeavours showcased a commitment to a healthcare system that values, honours and caters to the needs of all clients, irrespective of their background. Aisha's achievements were a powerful testament to the importance of embracing diversity and cultural understanding in healthcare. Her profound influence contributed to advancing a fair, empathetic, and inclusive healthcare system for everyone.

Aisha's diversity program focused on creating an inclusive environment where clients from diverse backgrounds felt appreciated and empathised. She successfully established client advisory councils that included representatives from diverse communities through her actions. These councils provided valuable perspectives and contributions, helping shape policies and procedures prioritising inclusivity and client-centeredness.

The success of her program ignited a broader conversation about the importance of diversity and inclusivity within the healthcare community. Aisha's research showcased the significance of understanding and addressing the unique needs of every client, leading to enhanced health outcomes and more efficient care.

Aisha fostered relationships with educational institutions to promote opportunities in healthcare for students from underrepresented backgrounds, driven by her commitment to fostering diversity. Partnerships with Mercy Mwongozo Hospital offered valuable opportunities and support to students, opening doors to careers in healthcare that they may not have considered otherwise.

Aisha recognised the importance of language in delivering comprehensive care. She expanded the hospital's translation services and introduced a program to educate employees on basic medical terminology in various languages. This endeavour contributed to eliminating language barriers, guaranteeing that every client could effectively communicate with their healthcare providers and receive the necessary care.

Aisha's program had a far-reaching impact that extended beyond the confines of the hospital. It began to influence municipal health policies, increasing community-based health initiatives targeting underprivileged and marginalised individuals. Her work has inspired other healthcare organisations to address health inequities and foster an inclusive environment proactively.

Aisha's story in her diversity program is a testament to the profound impact of unwavering commitment, compassion, and a deep grasp of the community. Her journey showcased the wide-ranging impact of advocating for and implementing diversity and inclusion in healthcare.

Aisha's initiatives continued to inspire and guide, setting a new standard for delivering comprehensive and equitable healthcare. Her work exemplified a commitment to a healthcare system that promotes inclusivity and dignity for all clients while addressing their medical needs. Aisha's achievements served as a powerful reminder of the vital role that healthcare providers play in fostering a more inclusive, empathetic, and compassionate world. Through her unwavering dedication, she has ensured that the impact of her diversity program will endure, leaving a lasting impression on healthcare for generations to come.

Aisha's impressive achievements in her diversity program sparked a wave of innovative community health initiatives. Realising that health disparities often stemmed from broader societal factors, she took proactive steps to tackle the social determinants of health head-on. Aisha prioritised nutrition, housing, and education programs, recognising the importance of combating these areas for sustainable health outcomes.

Her dedication to community health led to establishing health education centres in various neighbourhoods, especially those lacking adequate resources. These centres provided multiple resources, classes, and support on different health subjects, from managing chronic diseases to ensuring healthy pregnancies. They transformed into centres of knowledge and empowerment, vital in enhancing the community's understanding of health and promoting awareness.

Aisha recognised the importance of mental health and how it can affect one's overall well-being. She integrated mental health services into her diversity program, offering culturally sensitive counselling and support groups. This endeavour contributed to destigmatising mental health care and enhancing its accessibility for individuals who may have been reluctant to seek assistance otherwise.

Aisha is dedicated to broadening access to care in her efforts to create a more inclusive healthcare system. She collaborated with local clinics to extend their operating hours and expand their range of services. Additionally, she advocated for policy reforms that improved healthcare access for marginalised individuals. Her diligent work ensured that more individuals received the necessary care promptly.

The impact of Aisha's diversity program started to influence the curriculum of medical and nursing schools. Understanding the importance of equipping healthcare workers with cultural competence and sensitivity towards diversity, educational institutions have begun integrating these topics into their curricula. Aisha's techniques and methods were utilised as case studies to educate future healthcare practitioners on the significance of inclusivity and respect in client care.

Aisha's work has generated additional interest in studying health inequalities and the efficacy of diversity programs. She collaborated with researchers to investigate the effects of her programs, contributing to the expanding collection of evidence highlighting the significance of diversity and inclusivity in healthcare. This study validated Aisha's work and offered guidance for other institutions looking to adopt similar programs.

Aisha's remarkable achievements in her diversity program have continued to ignite motivation and drive for transformation. Her story vividly showcased the power of one individual's determination and insight to improve healthcare and the community's overall welfare.

Aisha's endeavours have persistently been shaped and directed, serving as an exemplar for establishing a more comprehensive and equitable healthcare system. Her work showcased a solid commitment to promoting equal access to a healthy life for all individuals, regardless of their background. Aisha's achievements highlighted the importance of acknowledging and embracing diversity in all areas of healthcare. Her unwavering dedication to this cause ensured that the principles of her diversity program would persist and bring about transformation, driving advancements toward a healthcare system that genuinely caters to everyone.

Aisha's program gained recognition as a prime example of how healthcare systems can effectively address the needs of diverse populations and provide top-notch care. She started supporting local governments and health departments in crafting and executing policies that tackled health disparities and fostered a more inclusive healthcare setting.

She additionally developed a comprehensive guide for healthcare providers, offering practical steps and valuable resources to enhance their understanding and integration of diversity and inclusivity principles into their professional practice. This toolbox was widely distributed, becoming an invaluable resource for healthcare practitioners seeking to customise their care to the needs of diverse communities.

Aisha's contributions influenced the overall client experience. Clients started sharing anecdotes about feeling acknowledged, heard, and valued in ways they hadn't experienced previously. These stories showcased the power of a healthcare system that values every individual's background, convictions, and needs. They also inspired other healthcare practitioners to follow in Aisha's footsteps.

As her program gained more recognition, Aisha received partnership offers from international health organisations. She dedicated her efforts to global projects to address health inequities and foster inclusivity in global healthcare systems. Her expertise and background have contributed to the worldwide pursuit of health equity.

The narrative of Aisha's achievements in her diversity program unravelled as a remarkable story of commitment, creativity, and compassion. Her journey showcased the extensive impact of healthcare initiatives, emphasising inclusivity and respect for diversity.

Aisha's initiatives have consistently sparked inspiration and provided valuable guidance, setting a fresh standard for the operation of healthcare systems. Her work exemplified a commitment to a healthcare system that promotes not only the treatment of illnesses but also fosters respect, understanding, and equality. Aisha's achievements served as a powerful reminder of the vital role that healthcare providers play in promoting a more inclusive, empathetic, and fair society. Through her unwavering dedication, she ensured that the legacy of her diversity program would have a lasting impact on healthcare, making a significant difference in the lives of countless individuals for years to come.

CHAPTER 36

Miriam's Resolution

Miriam, a highly analytical and creative Mercy Mwongozo Hospital healthcare expert, significantly integrated cutting-edge technologies into client care. He deeply understood the moral dilemmas that often accompanied advancements in science. His mission transformed into a pursuit of finding a harmonious equilibrium between leveraging technology to enhance healthcare and upholding the ethical principles that form the foundation of the medical field.

He assembled a diverse council of healthcare professionals, ethicists, and technology experts from various fields. The committee's objective was to develop recommendations for the ethical use of technology in healthcare. These guidelines highlighted the importance of human supervision in therapeutic decisions, client consent, and confidentiality.

Miriam highlighted the significance of transparency in the utilisation of technology. He strongly advocated for transparent communication with clients regarding using technology in their healthcare and the potential impact on their treatment. This level of openness facilitated the cultivation of trust and guaranteed that clients remained the focal point of care decisions.

He also arranged workshops and seminars for healthcare staff to teach them the ethical considerations of using technology in the healthcare environment. During these sessions, participants were encouraged to explore various situations and case studies, prompting them to analyse and consider the responsible and ethical use of technology.

Miriam found the application of artificial intelligence (AI) in diagnosis and treatment planning particularly fascinating. He dedicated his efforts to developing AI systems that prioritise accuracy and efficiency while implementing mechanisms to identify and rectify potential biases. Consequently, the AI systems ensured all clients received fair and equal care.

Miriam's contributions started to influence the hospital's perspective on technology. After thoughtful deliberation of their ethical ramifications, decisions regarding integrating new technologies were made. The staff felt a heightened sense of confidence in utilising technology in manners that aligned with their dedication to client well-being.

Miriam's unwavering commitment to finding a harmonious intersection between ethical considerations and scientific progress led to a robust client advocacy program. This program prioritised considering client rights and preferences when implementing new technologies in care.

Miriam's work at Mercy Mwongozo Hospital exemplifies a remarkable story of foresight, responsibility, and creativity. It showcases his ability to navigate the complex intersection of ethics and technology. His journey highlights the importance of ethical considerations in the rapidly evolving realm of healthcare technology.

Miriam's activities have consistently served as inspiration and guidance, setting a remarkable example for healthcare organisations on effectively navigating the intricate relationship between technology and ethics. His work exemplified a commitment to a healthcare system that embraces technological advancements while also upholding the ethical values that form the foundation of client care. Miriam's dedication was an impressive homage to the promise of a technologically advanced and morally upright healthcare future. His unwavering dedication to this equilibrium ensured that as healthcare progressed, it did so with a focus on both ingenuity and ethical principles.

Miriam's decision to reconcile ethical considerations with technological innovation ignited a heated debate within the healthcare profession. His insights and educational sessions made a difference at Mercy Mwongozo Hospital and other institutions grappling with the challenges of modern healthcare technology. He gained recognition as a highly regarded speaker and consultant, generously imparting his expertise and knowledge to a broader audience while championing the importance of ethical standards in adopting technology.

His activities also caught the attention of healthcare professionals in ethical education. Medical and nursing schools recognised the importance of ethics training and included comprehensive instruction in their curricula. This ensured that future healthcare providers would be fully prepared to navigate the complex ethical landscape of a technologically advanced society.

Miriam acknowledged the ever-changing nature of technology and the necessity for ethical rules to adapt accordingly. He implemented a continuous review process for the recommendations to ensure their continued relevance and effectiveness in light of new developments. This process involved collecting regular feedback from healthcare professionals, clients, and technology experts to develop a dynamic and responsive ethical framework.

In addition, Miriam emphasised the importance of involving clients in discussions regarding healthcare technology. He established forums and feedback sessions to provide clients with a platform to share their stories and voice their concerns. Ensuring clients' direct engagement ensured that their voices and opinions played a vital role in the technology and ethics discussion.

Miriam's work had a profound influence that extended beyond individual client care. His unwavering commitment to finding a harmonious blend of ethics and technology was pivotal in fostering a thoughtful and morally conscious approach to advancing healthcare innovation. It ignited a culture of ethical responsibility that highly valued client welfare, transparency, and fairness.

Miriam's story compellingly illustrates the crucial role of ethical considerations in guiding technological advancements in healthcare. His journey highlighted the vital significance of taking a proactive and intentional approach to incorporating new technologies into client care.

Miriam's endeavours have had a lasting impact, serving as a model for ethical accountability in healthcare technology. His work exemplified a commitment to a healthcare system that strives for progress and innovation, all while remaining conscious of its moral obligations. Miriam's unwavering commitment highlighted the importance of prioritising human values in healthcare. It emphasised the need for the sector to progress with empathy, consideration, and an uncompromising commitment to doing what is morally correct for clients. Through his tireless dedication, he ensured the ongoing discussion surrounding the intersection of technology and ethics in healthcare, paving the way for harmonious coexistence.

Miriam's endeavours contributed to establishing a fresh healthcare paradigm that prioritised enhancing the human aspects of care through technology rather than solely focusing on efficiency. He worked closely with technology developers, urging them to prioritise ethical considerations. This collaboration led to the development of user-friendly and client-centred technologies that not only met the moral standards of healthcare providers but also enhanced the quality of client care.

As his program progressed, Miriam's attention was directed toward the concept of informed consent within technology. He developed comprehensive guidelines to ensure clients received thorough information regarding the technology used in their care and its implications for their treatment and privacy. This approach empowered individuals by giving them a say and options in their care while ensuring that technology was utilised, honouring their independence and self-respect.

Miriam also acknowledged the immense potential of technology in addressing healthcare disparities. He spearheaded programs that utilised technology to provide high-quality treatment to marginalised and remote populations, overcoming barriers to access. These projects used telemedicine, mobile health applications, and other technologies to provide care in areas that lacked access, showcasing the potential of technology to promote fairness and righteousness in healthcare when guided by ethical principles.

Miriam's accomplishment led to the establishment of a global partnership that addresses ethical concerns in healthcare technology. This international consortium brought together healthcare professionals, ethicists, technologists, and client advocates to exchange best practices, address challenges, and showcase innovations. Miriam's involvement in this consortium significantly promoted a global agenda focused on the responsible utilisation of technology in healthcare.

His efforts significantly influenced regulatory organisations and healthcare theories. Driven by Miriam's rules and the tangible benefits they offered, legislation was enacted to ensure healthcare technology's ethical and responsible use. This legislation laid the groundwork for healthcare facilities to embrace technology morally soundly and prioritise clients' well-being.

Miriam's work has always been a source of inspiration, showcasing his visionary mindset, unwavering dedication, and significant impact. His experience showcased the profound influence that thoughtful, ethical thinking can wield over the future of healthcare technology and innovation.

Miriam's initiatives continued to inspire and guide, setting a benchmark for the seamless integration of technology into healthcare. His work exemplified a deep commitment to a future where technology in healthcare is utilised as an extension of the caregiver's dedication to client well-being, prioritising it over mere convenience or efficiency. Miriam's resolution showcased the potential of a cutting-edge healthcare system that prioritises ethics and client well-being. His steadfast dedication ensured that as healthcare technology progressed, it did so with a solid ethical basis, prioritising client care, dignity, and fairness.

Miriam's influence became evident not just in healthcare but also in the broader realm of technological advancement. Tech firms eagerly sought his counsel and expertise in developing innovative healthcare technology, ensuring that their products were at the forefront of the industry, aligned with ethical principles, and focused on clients' needs. By collaborating with these companies, he created technologies prioritising clients' needs and rights, setting new standards for ethical technology development in the industry.

In addition, Miriam's endeavours inspired a fresh wave of healthcare professionals who shared his dedication to harmonising technology and ethics. He became a mentor to many others, generously sharing his knowledge and wisdom and fostering a culture of ethical mindfulness in healthcare. Miriam played a significant role in shaping the future of the profession. He did this by delivering insightful lectures, publishing influential works, and providing valuable one-on-one mentoring. His efforts aimed to ensure that the upcoming generation of healthcare providers would uphold the values of ethical treatment in an ever-evolving technological landscape.

Miriam also recognised the importance of global cooperation in maintaining ethical standards in healthcare technology. He worked alongside international health organisations to establish global standards for the ethical use of technology in healthcare. These principles helped establish a global practice standard, ensuring that clients worldwide could benefit from technological advancements while safeguarding their rights and dignity.

As Miriam's work gained more recognition, he started exploring the potential of upcoming technologies like genomics, nanotechnology, and artificial intelligence in healthcare, with a strong focus on ethical integration. He organised discussions and brainstorming sessions, gathering experts from various fields to predict upcoming challenges and develop plans to tackle them, emphasising ethical standards in healthcare advancements.

Miriam's narrative flourished into a formidable movement that revolutionised healthcare technology. His journey became a powerful representation of the importance of ethical responsibility, showcasing how a commitment to ethics and the well-being of clients can shape the direction of technological progress.

Miriam's endeavours have consistently inspired and significantly shaped the future, setting a high standard for ethical excellence in healthcare. His work exemplified a commitment to a healthcare system that harnesses the power of technology while upholding its core ethical obligations. Miriam's resolution highlighted the vital significance of maintaining equilibrium, forward-thinking, and moral consciousness in an era of swift technological advancements. Through his unwavering dedication, he paved the way for a future in healthcare where a harmonious blend of innovation and ethics would prevail. This vision would lead to technology enhancing humanity's health, dignity, and overall well-being.

CHAPTER 37

Zara's Triumph

Zara, a formidable healthcare leader at Mercy Mwongozo Hospital, has always been dedicated to instigating transformative shifts in healthcare policy. With a deep understanding of the healthcare system's intricacies and constraints and an unwavering commitment to client well-being, she became a strong advocate for significant policy enhancements. Her pursuit symbolises the profound impact of activism and visionary thinking on healthcare.

From the start, she prioritised enhancing client access to top-notch care. Zara started her research by conducting thorough analysis and gathering data to identify the shortcomings and inefficiencies in the current healthcare system. Equipped with compelling evidence, she organised meetings with lawmakers, healthcare providers, and client advocacy organisations to engage in discussions and devise comprehensive policy reform strategies.

Zara's primary objective was to advocate for policies that supported proactive treatment and timely intervention. She understood the importance of preventing or detecting illness early, which could significantly reduce healthcare costs and enhance client well-being. Her diligent work led to increased funding for community health programs, screenings, and public health education.

Zara dedicated significant efforts to address disparities in healthcare accessibility and improve its quality. She passionately supported legislation that aimed to eliminate obstacles to care, including high fees, insufficient insurance coverage, and geographical isolation. Her efforts contributed to the expansion of healthcare coverage and the construction of healthcare facilities in underserved communities.

Zara highlighted the importance of prioritising client-centred care to bring about policy change. She advocated for regulations that mandate healthcare systems to involve clients in care decisions, ensuring that treatment plans align with medical standards and clients' interests and values.

Zara's commitment to improving healthcare policy extended far beyond her local community. She collaborated with national and international health organisations, exchanging knowledge and gaining insights from global best practices. Her work started to significantly impact broader aspects of healthcare policy, leading to extensive reforms.

Zara's impactful contributions to major healthcare policy reforms at Mercy Mwongozo Hospital and other institutions have created a compelling narrative of solid leadership, effective lobbying, and significant impact. Her journey showcased how dedicated individuals can significantly impact intricate systems.

Zara's endeavours persistently stimulate and direct, establishing a clear understanding of the role of a healthcare advocate. Her efforts showcased a commitment to a fair healthcare system, focused on the client, and adaptability to all needs. Zara's triumph showcased the power of foresight, determination, and collaborative efforts in reshaping healthcare policy. Her ongoing impact led to significant advancements in the healthcare system, resulting in improved accessibility, quality, and treatment for all clients.

Zara's impact on healthcare policy resonated across the government and healthcare industries. Through her inclusive approach, she successfully brought together a diverse group of stakeholders, including clients, healthcare workers, lawmakers, and insurance firms, each offering unique insights into the conversation. This coalition collaborates to achieve similar objectives, dismantling outdated barriers and promoting a comprehensive approach to healthcare reform.

Her persistent advocacy also led to increased transparency in healthcare policy decisions. Zara supported holding open forums and public hearings to allow community members to voice their concerns and participate in policy discussions. This level of openness and transparency fostered a sense of trust among the public, guaranteeing that policies were aligned with the community's desires and requirements.

Zara emphasised the importance of integrating research and data into the legislative process to ensure that healthcare decisions were made with the utmost reliance on the best available evidence. She worked closely with academic institutions and research organisations to analyse intricate health data and provide actionable policy recommendations. This approach, grounded in research and analysis, led to improved policies that had measurable impacts on client care and outcomes.

Zara's study highlighted the importance of adaptability and flexibility in healthcare policy. She advocated for policies that could be readily adjusted in light of new evidence, emerging health risks, or evolving social needs. Thanks to its flexibility, the healthcare system stayed nimble and robust amid change.

Zara started guiding the upcoming cohort of healthcare executives as her successes in advocating for healthcare policies increased. She shared her expertise and wisdom, inspiring others to drive policy change and equipping them with the necessary resources and strategies to become impactful advocates. Zara was committed to leaving a lasting impact through her mentorship, advocating for a future where healthcare policy continually strives for fairness, effectiveness, and empathy.

Zara's story unfolded as a compelling illustration of how dedicated, unwavering advocacy can result in significant advancements in healthcare. Her journey showcased the considerable impact that dedicated individuals can make in shaping policies that impact the health and overall welfare of entire communities.

Zara's endeavours remained a source of inspiration and guidance, establishing a solid foundation for forthcoming alterations in healthcare policies. Her endeavours showcased a commitment to a healthcare system that addresses present needs and anticipates and adjusts to future challenges. Zara's triumph highlighted the significance of activism, collaboration, and empirical data in shaping a fairer, more efficient, and more empathetic healthcare system. Her unwavering dedication ensured that pursuing enhanced healthcare policy would remain a vital and influential factor in advancing healthcare for all.

Zara's dedication to healthcare policy reform ignited a transformation in how healthcare systems valued and embraced input from clients and communities. She developed systems and programs that facilitated more consistent and structured client feedback, ensuring that the perspectives of those directly impacted by healthcare policies were acknowledged and considered. This transition facilitated the formulation of more equitable and effective policies, as they were grounded in clients' real-life experiences and requirements.

Her research emphasised the importance of collaboration across different sectors in healthcare policy. Zara understood that various elements, such as education, environment, and socioeconomic circumstances, impacted health. She reached out to leaders in different fields, encouraging them to collaborate to tackle the broader factors influencing health. This approach led to the development of more comprehensive and practical health policies that acknowledged and attacked the intricate network of health-related factors.

Zara is dedicated to tackling health disparities marginalised communities face in her quest for equal healthcare. She championed policies that focused on the unique requirements of these populations, including improved availability of healthcare services, customised health education programs, and enhanced funding for community health initiatives. Her efforts contributed to narrowing the disparities in health outcomes among different communities, leading to a more fair and comprehensive healthcare system.

Zara's global impact extended to the international stage, where she partnered with global health organisations to advocate for and implement her effective policy measures in other countries. Her extensive collaboration contributed to the widespread adoption of effective healthcare techniques and policies, enhancing global health outcomes.

As Zara's influence as a policy champion grew, she started using her platform to advocate for increased and sustained investment in healthcare. She dedicated her efforts to improving public health, research, and healthcare infrastructure funding. Her initiatives highlighted the importance of prioritising long-term investments in health, ensuring that healthcare systems are adequately equipped to provide top-notch care and effectively address future challenges.

Zara's work story remains a testament to her passion, determination, and significant influence. Her experience underscored the power of advocacy and foresight in bringing about meaningful transformations in healthcare policy.

Zara's activities have consistently been a source of inspiration and have played a significant role in shaping the future. They have set a new benchmark for what it entails to be a healthcare policy advocate. Her work demonstrated a commitment to a just, adaptable, and progressive healthcare system. Zara's triumph was a powerful reminder of the importance of persistent advocacy, teamwork, and intelligent decision-making in crafting policies that enhance healthcare for all. Her steadfast dedication ensured that the movement towards improved healthcare policy would remain a crucial and vibrant force, consistently advocating for a fairer, more efficient, and empathetic healthcare system.

Zara's work profoundly impacted the educational framework for healthcare professionals. She emphasised the importance of understanding and shaping healthcare policy from the beginning of their careers. As a result of Zara's impressive accomplishments, educational institutions started integrating policy studies into their healthcare curricula. Consequently, a new wave of healthcare professionals has emerged, armed with clinical skills and a comprehensive understanding of the healthcare policies that shape their profession and the well-being of their clients.

Zara's advocacy efforts were widely recognised as a model for policy reform that prioritises clients' needs. Her impact on education was also highly regarded. She has convincingly demonstrated that involving clients and comprehending their needs can improve healthcare policy more effectively and sustainably. Hospitals and healthcare organisations worldwide adopted similar techniques, implementing their client advocacy and feedback systems inspired by Zara's successful models.

Through her unwavering commitment to promoting fair and accessible healthcare policies, she successfully spearheaded the creation of multiple support networks and coalitions. These networks united individuals from diverse backgrounds, including clients, healthcare practitioners, and advocates, to effect positive healthcare policy changes. They worked together to identify obstacles, offer remedies, and advocate for reforms that would enhance the accessibility, fairness, and efficiency of healthcare for everyone.

Zara's commitment to healthcare reform led her to explore innovative financial methods that could uphold and maintain equitable healthcare systems. She collaborated with economists, policymakers, and healthcare experts to create funding mechanisms to ensure quality healthcare for all rather than a select few. Her research highlighted the importance of sustained financial investment in achieving long-term healthcare objectives.

Zara's achievements in healthcare policy continued to shine as a remarkable testament to the influence of well-informed and passionate advocacy. Her journey inspired others, showcasing the power of commitment, teamwork, and a deep comprehension of the obstacles to bring about significant and lasting changes in the healthcare system.

Zara's endeavours have persistently steered and motivated others in their quest for an improved healthcare system. Her work exemplified a commitment to a future where the needs and voices of clients shape healthcare policy, professionals act as advocates in addition to carers, and healthcare is recognised as a fundamental right for everyone. Zara's triumph showcased the enduring influence of lobbying and the potential to establish a fairer, more efficient, and empathetic healthcare system through unwavering dedication and knowledge. Her steadfast commitment led to ongoing advancements and breakthroughs in healthcare policy, prioritising the welfare of clients as the focal point of healthcare.

CHAPTER 38

Breaking the Stigma

John, a caring and progressive healthcare provider at Mercy Mwongozo Hospital, had always been concerned about the negative perception surrounding mental health. He witnessed firsthand the obstacles that this stigma created for individuals seeking assistance and its impact on their healing and overall quality of life. John embarked on a series of mental health programs, driven to change their perspective significantly.

He began by coordinating hospital-wide training courses that focused on enhancing understanding of mental health, identifying signs of mental illness, and responding with empathy and sensitivity. These seminars gave healthcare personnel valuable insights into mental health issues, debunked misconceptions, and fostered a supportive and empathetic environment for clients and staff.

John also implemented a peer support program within the hospital. This program connected individuals with mental health challenges with others navigating similar experiences, fostering a network of support, empathy, and shared knowledge. The peer support program became a central focus of John's activities, highlighting the significance of understanding and collective experience in addressing the sense of detachment that can be associated with mental illness.

Appreciating the significance of increased community engagement, John initiated several public awareness initiatives. These initiatives utilised various media for communicating stories, facts, and information about mental health, aiming to educate the public and promote open conversations about mental illness. The campaigns also provided valuable information about available options and support, making it more convenient for individuals to seek assistance.

John's endeavours also focused on healthcare practitioners' well-being and mental health. He acknowledged the significant levels of stress and burnout they often faced and introduced initiatives within the hospital to provide mental health support. Programs offered included counselling services, stress management courses, and initiatives to enhance work-life balance. John fostered a more nurturing and compassionate environment for staff and clients by attending to the needs of the carers.

As it gained momentum, it started influencing policies and procedures beyond Mercy Mwongozo Hospital. Other healthcare organisations admired John's initiatives as a model for addressing mental health stigma in their organisations and communities. His work ignited a broader movement towards embracing more inclusive, empathetic, and nurturing methods in mental health.

John's work at Mercy Mwongozo Hospital to challenge the misconceptions surrounding mental illness unfolded as a remarkable tale of empathy, innovation, and advancement. His journey showcased the profound impact that understanding, encouragement, and meaningful conversations can have on mental health care and the individuals affected by mental illness.

John's endeavours were a source of inspiration and guidance, setting a new standard for how healthcare systems address mental health concerns. His work showcased a solid commitment to a future where mental health is recognised, stigma eradicated, and everyone has equal access to care and support. John's triumph was a remarkable testament to the potential of cultivating a more empathetic and inclusive approach to mental health care, guaranteeing that nobody endures in silence or shame. His unwavering dedication ensured ongoing advancement and optimism in the fight against the negative perception surrounding mental health.

John's ideas sparked widespread discussions and initiatives in the healthcare community, extending far beyond the boundaries of Mercy Mwongozo Hospital. He collaborated with schools, companies, and community organisations to expand his mental health awareness programs, reaching a wider audience and promoting a deeper understanding of mental health concerns.

He also established partnerships with mental health nonprofits and advocacy organisations. These collaborations helped to spread his message and offered additional resources and support for his endeavours. They collaborated on policy lobbying, advocating for policies that would enhance mental health services and reduce obstacles to care.

John understood the importance of continuous evaluation and improvement. He incorporated feedback systems into his programs to gain a deeper understanding of their effectiveness and identify areas for improvement. Receiving feedback directly from participants and clients was crucial in enhancing and broadening his projects to meet the community's needs.

His research also highlighted the importance of being culturally sensitive when addressing mental health concerns. John collaborated with cultural leaders and organisations to adapt his approach to maximise effectiveness and show respect. He ensured his programs were inclusive and considered diverse cultural perspectives on mental health.

John's efforts had a profound impact. Reports from both the hospital and the larger community indicate a shift in attitudes towards mental health. There was a noticeable increase in the number of individuals seeking care, with mental health discussions becoming more prevalent and accepted. The negative perception surrounding mental illness is gradually fading away.

The story of John's efforts evoked a vision of a world where mental health is openly discussed and effectively managed. His journey showcased the effectiveness of advocating, educating, and showing compassion in challenging and transforming the negative perception surrounding mental health.

John's actions have consistently inspired and motivated others in the ongoing battle against mental health stigma. His work demonstrated a commitment to a future where mental well-being is paramount, assistance is easily accessible, and no individual has to endure their struggles alone. John's accomplishment was a powerful reminder of the potential for change when dedication, knowledge, and compassion guide the path. His unwavering commitment ensured that the progress he initiated would be maintained, driving the movement to eradicate prejudice and foster a more compassionate and understanding approach to mental health for everyone.

John's studies started to influence the development of healthcare policies related to mental health on a larger scale. His efforts and their positive impact made a compelling argument for increased backing and resources for mental health services during his collaboration with legislators and healthcare experts. Through his dedicated work, he secured additional funding for mental health programs, expanded insurance coverage for mental health care, and bolstered resources for community-based mental health projects.

He highlighted the importance of early intervention and education in schools. John worked closely with educators to develop programs to educate children and teenagers about mental health. These programs focused on teaching them how to identify signs of mental distress in themselves and others and how to reach out for support. These programs aim to equip young individuals with the necessary knowledge and abilities to effectively manage their mental well-being and support their peers, leading to a future generation that is well-informed and empathetic.

John's activities also sparked increased research into mental health. Appreciating the importance of a deeper understanding of mental health disorders and more impactful treatments, he collaborated with research organisations. He provided funding for studies on different facets of mental health and care. This study provided valuable insights into mental health while dispelling myths and challenging preconceptions, reducing stigma even more.

John highlighted the significance of diverse treatment options in establishing a more comprehensive approach to mental health. He advocated for policies and practices that promoted a range of therapeutic approaches, ensuring individuals received personalised care tailored to their specific needs. Counselling, medical treatments, community support programs, and alternative therapies were discussed.

John understood the importance of caring for oneself and being resilient to maintain good mental health. He initiated wellness programs that focused on teaching stress management, mindfulness, and various coping techniques, empowering individuals to engage actively in their mental well-being. These programs highlighted the importance of prioritising mental well-being as a continuous journey, with the potential for everyone to make positive strides in their mental health.

As John's work gained more recognition, heartwarming stories started to surface about individuals whose lives were transformed by his initiatives. The personal testimonials added a profound and human element to the narrative of his work, showcasing the strong and positive impact that his efforts had on the lives of many.

John's work to end the stigma of mental illness has sparked a vision of a more compassionate, empathetic, and proactive approach to mental health care. His experience showcased the profound impact of dedication, support, and empathy in changing perspectives and improving care.

John's endeavours have persistently guided and motivated me, laying the foundation for a future where the significance of mental health is acknowledged as a vital aspect of overall well-being. His work exemplified a commitment to fostering a society that prioritises the well-being of its members' minds, ensuring that assistance is readily accessible and no one is left to battle mental illness in isolation. John's triumph was a powerful testament to the transformative potential of addressing mental health with mindfulness, compassion, and a dedication to making a difference. His unwavering commitment ensured that the drive to eliminate the social stigma surrounding mental health would persist, creating a society where mental well-being is acknowledged, valued, and supported by all individuals.

John's unwavering commitment to eliminating the negative perception surrounding mental illness led to the establishment of a comprehensive support system at Mercy Mwongozo Hospital. He created a wellness centre that provided a hub for staff and clients to access various resources, participate in training sessions, and receive essential mental health support. This centre became a sanctuary for many, symbolising the hospital's commitment to providing equal care and empathy for mental health as it does for physical health.

Appreciating the connection between mental and physical well-being, John made it his mission to seamlessly incorporate mental health care into the hospital's comprehensive healthcare services. He advocated for the inclusion of regular mental health screenings in routine medical check-ups, emphasising the importance of addressing mental health concerns alongside physical well-being. This integration facilitated the normalisation of mental health care and ensured that clients received a more comprehensive approach to their health.

John also understood the significance of fostering a sense of community to support mental well-being. He contacted local organisations, forming partnerships to create a support network beyond the hospital's confines. These community collaborations offered various resources and assistance to individuals facing mental health challenges, including counselling, support groups, employment aid, and housing assistance.

John advocated for open communication and storytelling to challenge the negative perceptions surrounding mental health. He orchestrated gatherings where individuals could share their personal or loved ones' encounters with mental illness. These stories help to bring a unique perspective to mental health challenges, fostering empathy and understanding within the community.

John's successful endeavours inspired other healthcare facilities to follow suit. His approach to integrating mental health care and addressing stigma has been replicated in different institutions and healthcare settings, expanding the impact of his work.

John's efforts to eradicate the negative perception surrounding mental illness served as a symbol of hope and advancement. His experience showcased the profound impact of empathy, creativity, and determination in reshaping perspectives and enhancing livelihoods.

John's efforts have been a source of inspiration and have had a significant impact, paving the path for a future where mental health is openly addressed, actively supported, and treated with the attention it deserves. His work exemplified a commitment to a society prioritising mental well-being and providing the necessary assistance and compassion to uphold it. John's triumph showcased the strength of empathy and action, even in the face of stigma and ignorance. His unwavering dedication ensured further advancements toward a society that genuinely embraces and uplifts mental well-being, leaving no room for hidden suffering or stigma.

CHAPTER 39

Grace's Golden Years

Grace, a seasoned and compassionate nurse at Mercy Mwongozo Hospital, has devoted her career to enhancing geriatric care. Her innovative approach prioritises improving the quality of life for older individuals by providing considerate, compassionate, and thorough care. Her program quickly gained recognition as a benchmark for senior care, setting fresh standards for how the healthcare system tackles the ageing population's needs.

Grace started by creating a holistic care model that catered to older individuals' physical, emotional, and social needs. She educated her colleagues to see beyond the apparent medical challenges, recognising that the welfare of elderly clients often hinged on a range of factors. Her team acquired the ability to identify the signs of loneliness, despair, and cognitive decline, which are equally crucial to address in elderly care as physical health concerns.

Grace's program highlighted the importance of empowering older individuals to choose their care, emphasising autonomy and dignity. She implemented care planning sessions to facilitate open communication between clients, their families, and their care providers, allowing them to discuss their preferences, goals, and concerns. This collaborative approach ensured the care aligned with the client's values and desires.

Grace also acknowledged the significance of the environment in senior care. She dedicated her efforts to enhancing the ambience and ensuring the utmost comfort in the hospital's geriatric ward. The award was thoughtfully redesigned, considering older people's needs. The layouts were simple, and the colours were chosen to create a soothing atmosphere. Additionally, spaces were designed to encourage social interaction and provide recreation opportunities. This environment enhanced the hospital experience for older clients and contributed to their overall well-being and recovery.

Grace developed a volunteer program that facilitated connections between community members and older individuals, addressing the social needs of elderly clients. These dedicated individuals accompanied the clients, shared meals, and participated in leisure activities. The program helped combat feelings of loneliness and isolation by providing emotional support and enriching the lives of older individuals.

Grace's pursuits extended beyond the hospital. She worked with community organisations to create support networks for older individuals who cannot leave their homes. These networks offered various services, such as health education, home health care, and assistance with daily tasks. Grace's program significantly improved the lives of older individuals by providing them with the necessary assistance to maintain their independence and enhance their overall well-being in the comfort of their homes.

Her program gained popularity, prompting other nursing facilities to view it as a model for geriatric care. Grace has been invited to speak at conferences and workshops, where she has presented her ideas and strategies for compassionate, all-encompassing care for older people.

Grace's geriatric care work at Mercy Mwongozo Hospital was exceptional. It showcased her compassion, resourcefulness, and admiration for older people. Her journey exemplified the profound influence that a dedicated and intentional approach to caregiving can have on the well-being of older adults.

Grace's initiatives continued to ignite inspiration and provide guidance, ushering in a fresh era of geriatric care. Her work exemplified a commitment to a healthcare system that offers the utmost respect, empathy, and comprehensive care that older individuals require. Grace's accomplishment was a powerful reminder of the importance of acknowledging and addressing the unique requirements of older people. Her unwavering dedication ensured that her legacy would endure, positively influencing the standard of geriatric care for years to come and guaranteeing that the later stages of life are experienced with honour, compassion, and happiness.

Grace's program started to influence national policy discussions significantly as her geriatric care model showed clear advantages not just for older people but also for the healthcare system as a whole. She played a crucial role in formulating policies that promoted the idea of older individuals staying in their homes, advocating for services that enabled them to maintain their independence for as long as possible.

Through diligent work, she secured additional funding for geriatric education and training programs, guaranteeing that healthcare professionals could provide exceptional care to older people. Grace understood the importance of having highly skilled individuals who could effectively handle the complex needs of elderly individuals. She dedicated herself to advocating for the significance of specialised training in geriatric care.

Grace broadened her program to incorporate technological solutions that enhanced the well-being and security of elderly individuals, alongside her efforts in policy and education. She collaborated with technologists to develop user-friendly devices and systems that supported health monitoring, medication management, and communication with healthcare practitioners and family members. These advancements enabled older individuals to remain independent while receiving the necessary care and support.

Grace also understood the importance of research in the progress of senior care. She collaborated with academic institutions to research her program's impact, resulting in valuable data contributing to the enhancement and advancement of aged care. This study has contributed to the senior care field by enhancing our understanding of best practices. It has also been crucial in developing evidence-based guidelines that other institutions can adopt.

As it grew and evolved, it became a beacon of optimism and progress in aged care. Tales of enhanced well-being, self-sufficiency, and personal growth echoed throughout Mercy Mwongozo Hospital and beyond. Grace's work inspired similar endeavours and a renewed focus on the excellence of senior care.

Grace's story continued to unravel as a testament to her unwavering commitment, resourcefulness, and profound admiration for older people. Her experience showcased the profound impact that comprehensive, compassionate care can have on the lives of older individuals.

Grace's endeavours persistently motivate and steer, forging a future where older people are regarded with dignity and honour. Her work demonstrated a commitment to a healthcare system that recognises and values the contributions of older individuals. Grace's triumph showcased the potential for profound change when we approach geriatric care with reverence, empathy, and a dedication to excellence. Her unwavering commitment held the promise of further advancements toward a future where the later stages of life are filled with vitality, joy, and top-notch support.

Grace's influence went beyond direct client care; her program introduced a comprehensive approach to ageing and senior health encompassing the entire community. She worked with local organisations to create public education programs highlighting the importance of proactive health planning, gaining knowledge about ageing, and accessing necessary services and support. These programs sought to empower older people, their families, and carers, creating a knowledgeable and supportive community network.

Her commitment to providing thorough care led to the establishment of interdisciplinary geriatric health teams. Doctors, nurses, therapists, social workers, and other professionals collaborated to offer a comprehensive and integrated approach to each client's care. This multidisciplinary approach became a cornerstone in ensuring that all aspects of an elderly individual's health and well-being were thoroughly examined and addressed.

Grace also became a passionate advocate for end-of-life care that respected the desires and dignity of older people. She highlighted the importance of advanced care planning and promoted open conversations about end-of-life wishes and decisions among clients, families, and healthcare providers. Her expertise in this field ensured that older individuals received care aligned with their preferences and desires, providing comfort and tranquillity during their last years.

Grace's program gained recognition and backing from national healthcare agencies and ageing organisations as its reputation grew. Her geriatric care strategy received widespread recognition for its innovative and compassionate approach, leading to grants and financing to expand and enhance her programs. Grace broadened her program by implementing it in multiple locations, reaching many older individuals and their families.

Headed attention has been given to research on ageing and geriatric care. Grace collaborated with scholars to examine the enduring impacts of her program on health outcomes, quality of life, and healthcare expenses. The research findings offered valuable insights into effective methods of caring for older people and played a crucial role in shaping the future of senior care.

The story of Grace's labour sparked a vision of a society that appreciates and provides for its elderly population. Her story exemplifies the profound impact of empathy, innovation, and perseverance in elderly care.

Grace's endeavours persisted in guiding and motivating, setting a fresh standard for elderly care. Her work exemplified a commitment to a future where older people are treated with respect and provided top-notch care. Grace's victory highlighted the potential for meaningful progress when we approach aged care with understanding, kindness, and a dedication to excellence. Her unwavering commitment ensured the ongoing progress of geriatric care, allowing seniors to experience their later years with dignity, comfort, and happiness.

Grace's work began to resonate with healthcare professionals and institutions worldwide, sparking international collaboration and exchange. She participated in global ageing conferences and forums, exchanging ideas and gaining insights from diverse cultures and systems. These connections broadened her program by providing fresh perspectives and methods that can be utilised to enhance aged care.

Her unique perspective on senior care started to influence the design of healthcare facilities. Architects and planners sought Grace's expertise in creating environments prioritising the safety, accessibility, and overall quality of life for older individuals. Walking trails, gardens, and communal spaces in these environments encouraged social interaction and physical activity, promoting a healthier and more joyful lifestyle for older people.

Grace's focus on community involvement led to establishing senior advocacy groups in the neighbourhood. Motivated by her endeavours, these groups actively engaged in healthcare discussions and policy development, ensuring that the perspectives and requirements of older individuals were acknowledged and considered. Their goal was to raise awareness about the challenges of elder care and push for policy reforms that would benefit more senior people.

The success also highlighted the importance of providing emotional and psychological support for older people. Grace broadened her program to include mental health treatments upon recognising the significance of mental well-being alongside physical well-being. Her teams consisted of experts in the field of geriatric mental health, including psychologists and counsellors. They assisted older individuals dealing with common issues such as depression, anxiety, and grief.

As the impact of Grace's work expanded, it became a beacon of hope and motivation for individuals passionate about senior care. Her journey showcased the profound influence that dedication, knowledge, and innovation can have on the well-being of elderly individuals.

Grace's innovative ideas revolutionised the senior care field, setting a new benchmark for excellence. Her work exemplified a commitment to a healthcare system that values and appreciates the inherent worth of every individual, regardless of age. Grace's triumph highlighted the importance of offering older individuals the care, respect, and dignity they are entitled to. Through her unwavering dedication, she ensured that the impact of "Grace's Golden Years" would endure, shaping the field of senior care and guaranteeing that older people are treated with empathy, exceptional care, and respect.

CHAPTER 40

A New Beginning in Nursing

A serene atmosphere filled the air as the first light of day graced Mercy Mwongozo Hospital. The characters gathered to discuss their adventures and the profound lessons they had learned, each embodying transformation and determination uniquely. This event was more than just a conference; it was a joyous commemoration of the transformations they had observed and contributed to in nursing.

Emma, who had personal experience with the rapid advancements in nursing technologies, shared how her initial apprehension transformed into admiration and support. She explored the delicate equilibrium between technology and human connection, underscoring that while advancements can assist with caregiving, the nurses' compassion and empathy form the essence of their profession.

Contemplating his encounters with global health crises, David shared his heightened understanding of the interconnectedness of health. Through his work experience, he understood that the responsibility for promoting health extended beyond borders and cultural boundaries, requiring collective effort from individuals and communities. He underscored the importance of worldwide unity and collaboration in addressing health concerns.

Lina, the mastermind behind the groundbreaking nursing education, emphasised the importance of continuous learning and flexibility. She highlighted the impact of her innovative teaching methods, revolutionising nursing education and instilling a lifelong passion for knowledge and personal development.

Aisha shared her endeavours to address the issue of diversity in healthcare with a warm smile. She shared captivating stories of enhanced inclusivity and empathy, emphasising the importance of recognising and managing all clients' unique experiences and requirements, which lie at the core of nursing.

Miriam, renowned for his ethical stance on technology, emphasised the importance of maintaining moral integrity amidst the rapid pace of innovations. He highlighted the importance of keeping a harmonious equilibrium between efficiency and empathy, guaranteeing that each technological progress is undertaken with meticulous ethical deliberation.

John, who has made significant contributions to reducing mental health stigma, shared his vision for a future where mental health receives the same level of attention and importance as physical health. He emphasised the necessity of support systems, honest communication, and fostering a culture of mental health awareness and care.

Grace, a compassionate leader in senior care, discussed the importance of upholding the dignity and respect of older people. She provided examples of transformed lives where older individuals were acknowledged and respected, with their wisdom and experience cherished by everyone.

Their stories were filled with a strong sense of resilience, adaptability, and a positive outlook. Every individual faced challenges and obstacles, yet their unwavering commitment and focus led to notable progress in nursing and healthcare.

We were focused on the collective journey of the nursing profession rather than the individual experiences of these individuals. It showcased the power of empathy, creativity, and determination. The event highlighted the novel's themes, reminding all present about the importance of advocating for others, continuously expanding our knowledge, and the compassionate aspect of nursing.

The conference concluded with a shared sense of hope and dedication. The characters and the entire Mercy Mwongozo Hospital staff played an active role in shaping and driving change. They were at the forefront of a new era in nursing, prepared to face the future with determination, optimism, and an unwavering dedication to enhancing the well-being of individuals. The journey ahead stretched before them, but they were well-equipped to face it. Their collective efforts made them committed to creating a lasting impact in nursing and healthcare.

The figures symbolised a distinct facet of healthcare evolution and recognised the obstacles ahead. Although significant advancements have been achieved, it is acknowledged that the journey of enhancement and adjustment is still in progress. Emma was committed to balancing innovation and traditional care, ensuring that advancements enhanced the essential human connection rather than replacing it.

David discussed his plans to become more involved in global health projects, realising that one community's health will unavoidably affect the larger tapestry of global wellbeing. He was dedicated to fostering cross-border collaboration to strengthen the international health community and enhance its resilience.

Lina discussed the future of nursing education with a contemplative nod. She imagined a society where every nurse would graduate with practical skills and knowledge, an insatiable thirst for knowledge, and deep compassion. She was determined to continuously explore and innovate in the field of education, embracing any necessary tools, theories, or methods to cultivate highly skilled and empathetic nurses.

Aisha discussed her future goals of expanding the reach of her programs, which have made significant strides in promoting diversity in healthcare. She aspired to extend her reach to additional underserved populations, providing awareness, support, and care to individuals who had previously been overlooked. She confidently stated that her mission was far from over; it expanded daily.

Miriam is committed to remaining vigilant and protecting at the intersection of innovation and ethics. He was steadfast in his ethical approach to advancing technology. He understood the importance of thoroughly evaluating every new development to uphold and enhance ethical standards.

John envisioned a future where mental health held a prominent place in healthcare, supported by advancements in reducing the stigma surrounding it. He imagined programs and policies that emphasised psychological and physical health. In this world, support was readily available, and the shame surrounding it was a thing of the past.

Grace envisioned a world where the golden years of life were genuinely golden, with a heart full of stories from older people she'd cared for. She imagined a world where senior care was associated with dignity, respect, and joy. Her dedication to improving the lives of older people was unshakable, and her goals were broad, promising continuing innovation and compassion.

These individuals, these catalysts for change, united in their shared vision for a brighter future in nursing and healthcare. They recognised that their travels were not isolated; they were part of a more remarkable story, a collaborative effort for better, more compassionate, and more effective healthcare. Their narratives continued to unfold, woven with strength, growth, and optimism. They were only beginning, with each new day offering a chance to grow, create, and motivate. Their unwavering commitment shone brightly, guiding the way towards a fresh era in nursing. This era held the promise of enhanced care, profound comprehension, and an everlasting quest for excellence in the noble cause of serving humanity.

The group celebrated the broader community of nurses, healthcare workers, and support personnel who played a vital role in their stories as they reflected on their shared experiences and individual contributions. They recognised that, as they stood as change agents, countless others worked diligently daily, often without recognition, to provide care, comfort, and healing. They engaged in a thoughtful conversation about acknowledging and assisting the often-overlooked individuals in healthcare.

Emma discussed the future, envisioning a healthcare system that seamlessly integrated technology while focusing on the human aspect at its core. She envisioned a world where nurses embraced technology to amplify their inherent compassion and empathy rather than relying on it as a crutch. She expected a moment when every client would experience the warmth of human care, supplemented by the accuracy and support of cutting-edge technology.

With a determined expression, David described his idea for a worldwide health network that would cross political and cultural boundaries to address common concerns. He imagined a future in which health emergencies were met with coordinated, worldwide responses, and resources and expertise were freely shared to combat dangers to human health. He pledged to enhance relationships and partnerships, ensuring that in the face of a health crisis, every community would receive the backing and resources of the global community.

Lina imagined a future where nursing education held a significant and esteemed position. She imagined institutions worldwide adopting her all-encompassing and immersive approach, resulting in a new generation of nurses with clinical competence, deep empathy, a strong voice for their clients, and a commitment to lifelong learning. She envisioned a world where every nurse possessed the capacity to lead, innovate, and motivate.

Aisha spoke with great enthusiasm about her ongoing mission to integrate diversity, equity, and inclusion into the very essence of healthcare. She envisioned a future where every individual could receive compassionate and culturally sensitive care regardless of background. She observed a society where the healthcare workforce mirrored the diversity of the communities it catered to, diverse perspectives were highly regarded, and a sense of belonging was fostered for all.

Ever the astute observer, Miriam expressed his expectations for a future in which an ethical advancement accompanies every technological improvement in healthcare. He portrayed a society where ethics were not overlooked but instead a crucial element of healthcare advancement. He imagined a healthcare system asking more than "Can we?" It also considered "Should we?" and "How can we do this correctly?"

With a compassionate smile, John described his vision of a society where mental health is no longer stigmatised and care is available. He envisioned a future where discussions about mental health were just as expected and ordinary as discussions about physical health, and seeking assistance was seen as a display of resilience rather than vulnerability. He imagined a future where everyone had the support and resources to sustain their bodily, mental, and emotional well-being.

Drawing from her wealth of experience caring for older people, Grace envisioned a future where the later stages of life were cherished and celebrated. She envisioned a future where older individuals could live with dignity, where their contributions were acknowledged, and where their wisdom was valued. She imagined a time when senior care went beyond mere health maintenance and focused on enhancing the happiness and satisfaction of one's later years.

The group experienced a revitalised sense of purpose and dedication as they discussed their aspirations for the future. They acknowledged that, although their contributions had sparked change, it would require many's combined determination and involvement to maintain and enhance this progress. They understood that the future they imagined was not just a daydream but a potential reality that required ongoing perseverance, commitment, and optimism.

Their conversation, a rich tapestry of wisdom, ambition, and determination, highlighted the novel's underlying messages of resilience, transformation, and optimism. It stood as a testament to the strength of passionate individuals and a constant reminder of the tasks that still lay ahead. They concluded their meeting with solid enthusiasm, prepared to carry on the path of progress and advancement in healthcare, driven by their unwavering dedication to their clients, their profession, and one another.

The group acknowledged the power of working together, fueled by their mutual commitment and the narratives they had crafted collectively. They discussed expanding their networks and interacting with healthcare professionals worldwide to share knowledge, tactics, and support. They envisioned a global knowledge exchange, where insights gained in one location could be shared and utilised in another. They sought to solve challenges in hospitals by drawing lessons from the experiences of others.

They explored the importance of continuous advocacy, of coming together to amplify their voices to advance the interests and rights of healthcare professionals and clients alike. They envisioned creating platforms where their collective experiences could shape legislation, foster innovation, and bring about lasting transformations in the healthcare system.

The committee also recognised the importance of educating the upcoming generation of healthcare professionals. They explored mentorship programs, internships, and scholarships that aim to inspire and empower young individuals entering the field. They envisioned a future where experienced experts would generously pass on their wisdom, passion, and commitment to the next generation.

They discussed the obstacles they anticipated encountering while sharing their aspirations: resistance to change, scarcity of resources, and the magnitude of the undertaking. Instead of feeling overwhelmed, they found motivation. They understood that the journey they were embarking on required unwavering determination, resilience, and unwavering focus on the goal ahead.

They understood that, although they had all contributed to starting the change, the accurate measure of their success would be the long-term impact and ongoing nature of their endeavours. They discussed building systems and structures that would endure, leaving behind a lasting legacy of progress and compassion that would thrive even after their contributions faded.

As the meeting concluded, a sense of camaraderie and direction permeated the room. They were coworkers and comrades in a single cause, allies for a common purpose. They departed the gathering together, united in their purpose, prepared to face any challenges that may come their way, fully aware of the more significant cause they were a part of.

Their narrative, encompassing its challenges, triumphs, and aspirations, reflected the broader tale of nursing and healthcare. It was a tale of individuals coming together to create an impact, minor deeds resulting in significant transformations, and the ceaseless quest for a more empathetic and improved world.

They went their separate ways, fully aware that the future of nursing was not just a far-fetched dream but a tangible reality that they were actively shaping through their client care, policy influence, and mentorship of young professionals. This began a new chapter in their story, filled with the potential for ongoing development, significant impact, and an unwavering pursuit of excellence in nursing.

The group's departure from the meeting signalled their unwavering commitment as they continued to pursue their shared goals. Each member returned with a fresh sense of duty and a motivated drive to achieve their personal and collective goals. They left a deeper understanding of how their small contributions played a part in the larger narrative of progress and development in the nursing field.

They resumed their duties and started implementing the ideas and plans they had discussed. They enthusiastically shared their thoughts and commitments with their networks, encouraging others to join them in their mission. The profound impact of their assembly extended across hospitals, clinics, and healthcare facilities, reaching far and wide.

Emma consistently integrated technology with a compassionate approach, guaranteeing that every advancement enhanced nursing care. Her approach became a paradigm for striking a harmonious balance between efficiency and empathy in integrating nursing technology.

David broadened his global health initiatives by establishing partnerships that provided assistance and expertise to underprivileged areas. His commitment to fostering a united health community led to the successful implementation of programs that profoundly saved lives and enhanced health outcomes worldwide.

Lina's innovative ideas had a lasting impact on the future of nursing education. Her methods were embraced by institutions worldwide, leading to a new wave of nurses equipped to tackle the challenges of modern healthcare with knowledge and empathy.

Aisha expanded her diversity initiatives, ensuring that healthcare is more inclusive and equitable. Her efforts led to significant advancements in policy and practice, guaranteeing that healthcare was available and adaptable for everyone.

Miriam was unwavering in his commitment to promoting ethical considerations in technological advancements. His diligent work ensured that healthcare stayed rooted in honest and empathetic principles as healthcare evolved.

John's efforts in mental health programs have consistently worked towards dismantling societal barriers and reducing the stigma surrounding mental illness. His initiatives and efforts brought significant focus and support to mental health care, positively impacting individuals' well-being and societal perspectives.

Grace's senior care program has been expanded to give older individuals the respect and care they deserve. Her work profoundly influenced legislation and procedures, guaranteeing that older people were treated with utmost respect and empathy.

The characters stayed connected as they advanced, supporting and collaborating on various projects. They regularly convened to exchange their successes, obstacles, and concepts. They were a catalyst for transformation in the nursing profession, a shining light of optimism and advancement.

The story of their journey became a source of inspiration for countless individuals. It showcased the strength of perseverance, teamwork, and unwavering dedication to enhance healthcare. It was the story of ordinary individuals who made extraordinary contributions in their professions and the global arena.

As the tale of their journey neared its end, it became clear that the change they had initiated was merely the start. The envisioned future, characterised by improved care, cutting-edge practice, and unwavering support for the nursing profession, was slowly but surely materialising. Their experience was a powerful reminder of the constant need for change, the importance of taking action, and the potential for optimism in healthcare. Their journey persisted, just like the journeys of numerous other healthcare professionals worldwide, all driven by the noble purpose of tending to, healing, and enhancing the lives of individuals.

www.ingramcontent.com/pod-product-compliance
Lightning Source LLC
Chambersburg PA
CBHW032045280526
45784CB00011B/2773